The Power of L

CW00539653

7 Effective Techniques on How to Stop
Overthinking the Past, Heal Emotional
Wounds, and (Finally) Enjoy the
Freedom You Deserve, without
Ruminating

Logan Mind

EMOTIONAL INTELLIGENCE
for Social Success

FREE DOWNLOAD: pxl.to/loganmindfreebook

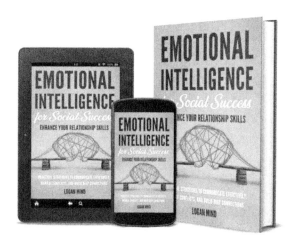

LOGAN MIND

EXTRAS

https://pxl.to/LoganMind

Books

Workbooks

FREE GIFTS

Review Team

Audiobooks

Contacts

CLICK NOW!

@loganmindpsychology

Download Your Free Book!

As a way of saying thanks for your purchase, I'm offering the **book** "Emotional Intelligence for Social Success" for **FREE** to my readers.

Inside this complimentary **guide**, you'll uncover **strategies** that can significantly improve your personal interactions and emotional skills. You'll learn about:

• Practical methods for improving emotional awareness

• Key techniques to enhance empathy and understanding

• Effective **communication** tips for any social situation

• Proven strategies for managing **stress** in relationships

• Ways to boost **confidence** through emotional intelligence

Unlock the potential of thriving social **engagements** by grabbing your free book today.

To get instant **access**, just head over to:

https://pxl.to/loganmindfreebook

How to Download Your Extras

Imagine getting the most out of this book with accessible resources that **boost** your progress every step of the way. Each extra can **amplify** your practice and understanding, making your path to emotional freedom not just easier, but more rewarding.

Here's what's waiting for you:

You'll get a downloadable and practical PDF 21-Day Challenge for the book that takes you through daily, actionable steps aimed at **solidifying** your learning and growth. Valued at $14.99, it turns the book's concepts into tangible actions, making implementation a breeze.

You'll also receive 101+ Mantras for Releasing Emotional Baggage, which give you **empowering** affirmations designed to shift your mindset. These mantras act as a mental reset button, helping you cut through the noise of overthinking.

The Emotional Regulation Essentials, worth $9.99, offers proven techniques for **mastering** your emotional responses. It teaches you skills that aren't just useful, but necessary for your overall well-being.

As a bonus, you'll get Emotional Intelligence for Social Success, worth $14.99 – a resource that **hones** your social skills and emotional intelligence, helping you navigate life's social complexities. Think of it as your ultimate cheat sheet for enhancing interactions and relationships.

By integrating these extras with the book, you'll be better **equipped** to make meaningful and lasting changes. Each of these tools has been carefully crafted to accompany and enrich your reading experience.

Check out the extras here:

https://pxl.to/7-tpolg-lm-extras

Other Books

Expanding your **knowledge** on related topics is key to truly letting go and finding peace. This book is a great starting point, offering you powerful techniques to stop overthinking the past, heal emotional wounds, and enjoy the freedom you deserve. But there's so much more to explore!

I've released several books, each targeting different yet interconnected aspects of emotional well-being. As you dive into this field, you'll find that gaining a broader perspective can boost your **growth** and improve every part of your life.

Imagine building on your newfound wisdom with a deeper understanding of **emotional agility**. This book helps you balance adaptability and resilience, crucial traits that enhance your journey towards emotional freedom. You'll also discover strategies to fight **emotional burnout**, ensuring you never feel swamped despite life's challenges. Plus, achieving emotional stability gives you the tools to maintain a rock-solid emotional foundation, guaranteeing lasting mental peace even when things get crazy around you.

Each book I've written builds on the principles and reinforces the practices from the others, creating a smooth path to all-around emotional health.

To check out the other books:

Head to the link below, click on "All My Books," and grab the ones that catch your eye. If you want to get in touch with me, you'll find all my contact info at the end of the link.

Check out all my books and contacts here: https://pxl.to/LoganMind

Join my Review Team!

Thank you for reading my **book**! Your support means the world to me. I'd love for you to join my **Review** team. If you're an avid **reader**, you'll have the chance to get a free copy of my book in exchange for your honest **feedback**. This would really help me improve my **writing** and share my stories with more readers.

Here's how you can join the ARC team:

• Click on the link or scan the QR code.

• Click on the book cover on the page that opens up.

• Click on "Join Review Team."

• Sign up on BookSprout.

• Get notified every time I release a new book.

You can **check** out the team here:

https://pxl.to/loganmindteam

Don't miss this **opportunity** to be part of an exciting **community** of readers and writers!

Introduction

Ever felt like you're walking around with a **backpack** full of rocks? We all carry **emotional** baggage from our past, and man—can it weigh us down! I've spent years of my life studying human behavior, digging into the **psychology** of why we cling to our regrets and hurts like we're never going to let go. That's why I wrote this book: I wanted to hand you the key to unlock **freedom** and peace. Trust me, the journey of letting go isn't easy, but it's worth it, and this is your roadmap.

You'll find I dive deep into how our minds work—the why behind the overthinking, the self-sabotage, and the **emotional** wounds that seem to fester forever. What's cool is, it's all laid out in simple, actionable steps. No jargon. No fancy theories. Just effective techniques.

Why is this important, you ask? Picture this: A life where you aren't bogged down by what others did to you, what you did wrong, or what could go south in the future. Imagine actually enjoying present moments without your mind wandering back to painful memories or over-anticipating worst scenarios. Sounds like a breath of fresh air, doesn't it? That's what emotional freedom feels like.

But let's not just talk about theory. How about a quick win right here? Think about a time when you were stuck in a rut, overanalyzing a past mistake. That cycle of "what-ifs" can paralyze you. What you'll find useful are these short practices designed to snap you out of such loops instantly. This isn't theory. These lessons are drawn from real-life applications, tested on countless individuals just like you.

Now, why listen to me? Great question. I've spent my career intertwining rigorous academic **knowledge** with down-to-earth practicality. My work with top-tier business minds and people going through personal crises has given me a 360-degree view of how tangled our emotions can get. Think of me less as a distant author and more like a guide walking beside you, dropping wisdom and practical solutions that you can apply right now.

Let's face it. Life's tough and people naturally avoid anything that promises change—why tamper with the storm you know? But resisting change only keeps you stuck. In this book, every chapter is a stepping stone towards overcoming the deeply ingrained fears, doubts, and judgments that keep you reliving your pain rather than learning from it and moving forward.

One common objection might be, "Won't ignoring the past make me reckless?" Ah, but see, it's the opposite. This book isn't about erasing your past. It's about acknowledging it, learning from it, and then setting yourself free from its grip. Here, you'll learn effective ways to assess your experiences and use them as stepping stones rather than shackles.

A pivotal thing you'll discover as you thumb through these pages: the power of small hits of progress. It's like learning to ride a bike; every wobble teaches you balance. The little exercises throughout are meant to make you aware of tiny victories that'll snowball into meaningful **change** over time. We build momentum together.

If I could make one final call to action, it'd be this: Give yourself the grace to redefine who you are without the burden of past judgments and constraints. Imagine stepping into a room without dragging in the ghosts of yesterday and wearing the armor of regret. Imagine how light you'd feel—to finally breathe easy. Well, isn't that something worth striving for?

So here's to getting started, to mastering the art of releasing what doesn't serve us, and finding the **freedom** to live our best lives. Stick with me. Dive in. Let's get those chains off. It's going to be quite the ride!

Chapter 1: The Fundamentals of Letting Go

Have you ever wondered why some **memories** cling to you like stubborn stains? I have—many times, actually. That's what this chapter is all about. By the time you reach the end, you'll start to feel ready to shed those past **burdens**. It's like that—I think and hope you'll agree.

Imagine facing those old **attachments** that keep you tangled up: the emotional grips, the endless overthinking. You'll discover clear ways to break free from them. Don't you want to feel lighter, less bogged down by yesterday's thoughts?

You'll dive into how your **brain** likes to hold on to things, even when they're not helpful. **Emotions** can be tricky, right? They pull at you in strange ways. We'll chat about that, too—not in a tough, complex way, but in a way that makes it all clear and practical.

Ever found yourself replaying an awkward **conversation** or a mistake over and over? In this chapter, you'll dig into why and get some real ways to quiet that noise. It's about finding some inner **peace**.

So, jump in. The emotional **freedom** you've been seeking? It's on the page ahead, with just the right mix of guidance and understanding. Ready? Let's go.

The Psychological Aspects of Releasing the Past

Your **brain** is like a massive library filled with all your experiences. Every **memory** sits on a shelf, some neatly organized and some just crammed in a corner. Holding onto old memories, especially bad ones, can mess up the whole organization. Suddenly, the memory of a bad breakup overlaps with an embarrassing moment at work. It's all mixed up. This mishmash doesn't just affect your shelves— it messes with your **mental health** too.

When old memories keep resurfacing, they drag you back to those emotional moments. You're not just recalling the fact; you're reliving the feeling. It's exhausting, and you might feel more anxious as a result. It's like you're stuck on an emotional treadmill, running but going nowhere. This constant loop can also mess with your sleep and zap your energy. You end up tired, frazzled, and worried about almost everything. Also, it becomes hard to focus on anything else going on now, because a part of you is stuck back then.

But hey, your brain's not stuck that way forever. It can change, kinda like remodeling that library. This idea, **neuroplasticity**, means your brain's capable of re-wiring itself. Pretty cool, right? Just like muscles flexing with exercise, thinking differently can help rewire your brain. Starting today, you can train it not to hold onto the past. It means forming new habits, like being mindful or using certain techniques to redirect your thoughts.

Let's say you keep thinking about an argument you had ages ago. Each time you let your mind wander, remind yourself of something positive instead. This helps redirect that mental energy. Slowly, those old pathways get less traffic and start to shut down. You'll find new paths in your "garden" growing, leading to thoughts that don't make you feel down all the time.

The mental perks of letting go? Oh, they're great. For one, less **anxiety**. Without those burdensome memories clouding your thoughts, you feel lighter—like a massive weight's been lifted. You'll also find it easier to manage your **emotions**. When you're not getting dragged back to sad or angry memories, you react better to stuff happening now. It's like shaking off old dust and finally seeing things clearly.

When you're not held back by old stuff, there's new room for **happiness**. You'll have more mental energy to invest in stuff that matters—better focus on work, more joy in your hobbies, stronger relationships. You aren't just finding a little more joy, you're also making new, happier memories. Those become the new books on your shelf.

It's not all sunshine and roses from day one. It takes effort, consistency, and some patience. But if you stick with it, you'll be amazed at how much better you feel. Over time, thinking differently will feel as natural as pulling on your favorite comfy sweater.

So, it's worth the effort. Every moment spent rethinking is a step towards a calmer mind and a happier, more relaxed you. Your brain's like the best friend you never knew you had, ready to help you write a better story on those shelves. Relax, adjust, and let your mental library be filled with brighter, newer **chapters**.

Identifying Attachment Patterns

You've probably heard of attachment theory, right? It's this **idea** that how you bonded with people as a kid affects how you connect with folks now. It's like the roots of a tree, going deep and influencing everything else. And this matters big time when you're trying to let go of past stuff. Why? Because the way you **attach** to people can make your emotional baggage stick around longer than an unwelcome houseguest.

Let's talk about some common attachment styles. They're like different categories your brain puts people into—safe, dangerous, unreliable. And trust me, this affects your ability to just let things go.

First up, there's the "secure" style. If you've got this, you're in luck. You probably find it easier to trust folks, get close, and let go of the old stuff. Your emotional closet isn't bursting at the seams like some others might be.

Then there's the "anxious" style. If this is you, you're often worried people will leave you. You might hold onto past hurts like they're treasures, replaying moments to figure out what went wrong, how you could've fixed it. Letting go? Feels impossible because you think you might lose something even more valuable.

Got the "avoidant" attachment style instead? You might be keeping everyone at arm's length. Past hurt acts like a shield—you think holding on keeps you safe from getting burned again. Relaxing your grip feels like you're lowering your defenses, which can be super scary.

Lastly, there's "fearful-avoidant." This one's the trickiest because it's like a mixed bag of the other styles. You want closeness but are scared of it. You try to push people away, but then feel lonely. Letting go can feel like you're sailing a ship without a map.

Now, how can you spot unhealthy attachment patterns? Easy. Think about your **relationships**. Do you find yourself clinging to people or pushing them away without a second thought? Banks of excuses probably form a wall between you and any deep connection. That wall isn't just keeping others out; it's keeping your old pain in. If you're always on high alert for betrayal or rejection, you're basically setting up camp in the past instead of moving forward.

Another sign: overthinking. When a tiny disagreement feels like the end of the world and you replay every word looking for hidden meanings, your past is sneaking into your present. That's unhealthy attachment, making you drag old wounds into new situations. It's like bringing dirty laundry on a dream vacation.

But how does all this mess with your personal **growth** and relationships? Simple—if you're holding onto old hurts, you're not giving yourself space to grow. It's like having a backpack full of rocks while trying to run a marathon. And relationships? They suffer too. If you're always fearful or overly clingy, you're not just hurting yourself—you're dragging others into your emotional whirlpool.

So what can you do? Start paying attention. Notice when past **experiences** creep into your mind and relationships. That's the first step to changing things. Just recognizing these patterns can make a big difference. And always remember—letting go isn't about forgetting the past; it's about knowing what to keep and what to let be.

In short, examining and understanding your attachment style isn't just an academic exercise. It's a practical step towards unburdening yourself from past emotional **baggage** and improving your present relationships. Recognize the unhealthy patterns, so you don't keep repeating the same mistakes. After all, life's complicated enough without us making it harder. And that, my friend, is the **power** of letting go.

The Role of Emotions in Letting Go

When you're trying to let go, **emotions** can act like those big, flashing highway signs. They tell you what's coming up, and if you need to take a different route. They either help you move forward or keep you stuck in traffic. When you feel anger, sadness, or regret, those are signs pointing back to something you haven't really worked through. If you ignore these signs, well, you end up driving in circles.

Now, that's where **emotional intelligence** comes in. What's that? Basically, it's just being good at noticing what you're feeling and knowing what to do about it. Sort of like being your own weather forecaster for your moods. It's important to know your emotional patterns—like, why do some past events still get under your skin? It's not just about figuring out that they irritate you; it's getting to the why and the how too. This makes a big difference. When you understand your own emotional weather, you're way better at staying balanced. No more sudden emotional downpours.

Think of emotions like visitors to your house. Some are pleasant, some... not so much. You don't always choose when they visit, but you do choose how long they stay and where they sit. **Managing** your emotions means deciding not to let the "bad" ones hang around too long. Yeah, easier said than done, right? But practice helps. It's all about feeling your feelings, but not becoming them.

So how does this connect to **letting go** of bad stuff from your past? Well, when you manage your emotions well, you're less likely to cling to that old hurt. Chances are, bad feelings have just settled in because they didn't get addressed at the time. When you recognize and deal with these emotions, you're cleaning house—making room for new, better feelings.

And sometimes, managing feelings is about having simple tools handy. Here are a few options:

• Deep breaths

• Going for a walk

• Journaling

These small actions can shift your mood and make it easier for you to handle those bigger emotional traffic jams.

But, here's an important bit—acknowledging emotions doesn't mean diving into them without a life jacket. It means catching them when they occur and then doing something constructive with that energy.

Take **sadness**, for example. It might stick around because you haven't given it enough attention. Think about grieving a past relationship. Let yourself feel sad, but also do activities that bring you joy. Slowly, that sadness loses its grip. Not because you ignored it, but because you handled it wisely.

Or consider **anger**. If not managed, it turns into bitterness, making it hard to let go of past grievances. It's like trying to drive with boulders in your trunk—it slows you down. Address the anger head-on. Perhaps by talking it out with someone or even through physical activity like a sport. Just make sure you're without those heavy rocks when you want to move forward.

In summary, your emotions are key players in the process of letting go. They shouldn't be locked away or ignored. Understanding them gives you insight into what still needs attention—sort of your own emotional GPS. By managing these emotional signposts, you make peace with the past and open up the road to finding the **freedom** you truly deserve.

And that's pretty much it. Handling emotions isn't just a part of letting go. It's the steering wheel guiding you to a better place.

Recognizing Overthinking and Rumination

Ever notice how **thinking** is a bit like driving? Sometimes, you cruise down the highway, enjoying the view and the journey itself. Other times, you hit the same stop sign over and over again, like you're trapped in a never-ending loop. That's the difference between simply thinking things over and getting stuck in **overthinking** or **rumination**.

Thinking things over can be productive. It's like mapping out a road trip. You consider your options, plan your stops, and ensure you're ready for what might come up. But overthinking? That's when your **brain** keeps circling around the same set of worries, playing out "what-ifs" and worst-case scenarios on repeat. You're not finding solutions anymore—you're just going in circles, stressed out, not getting anywhere.

Why does your brain do this? It's actually a survival mechanism. Your brain thinks it's helping. When you keep mulling over a problem, your brain is on high alert, looking for any potential danger or threat like a guard dog on duty. This made sense back when our ancestors had to worry about predators. But today? Well, it more often than not just makes you anxious. This high-alert state triggers your fight-or-flight response; once it's activated, it's really hard to switch off.

So, what comes from being stuck in these thought loops? For one, it messes with your **mental health**. Anxiety and depression can set in when your mind is always on guard, unable to let go of past mistakes or future fears. It's like being trapped in a fog that you can't escape from, making it really hard to see the good stuff around you.

Physically, it's not any better. Ever lie awake at night, your heart pounding, thinking about some minor thing and feeling like you just ran a marathon? Your body doesn't know the difference between real danger and imagined fears, so overthinking makes you feel like you're constantly under attack. This can lead to headaches, stomach issues, and weakened immunity making you more prone to getting sick. Your overall **energy** dips, too, as if you're running on an empty tank.

It's quite the mess, right? Stuck in a never-ending cycle of **stress** thinking you'll magically solve anything just by worrying more about it. But, stepping back makes it easier to see things with clarity and discern whether the problem is worth this energy in the first place.

Breaking free isn't easy given how sneaky these loops can be. Sometimes, they disguise themselves as problem-solving when really, they're just procrastination. You feel like you're making progress—going over the same material just one more time—but you're really just loitering around without doing anything constructive. The trick is figuring out when your thinking is productive and when it's just run-of-the-mill rumination.

So, what should you do? It all starts with **awareness**. You must catch yourself in the act. If you notice your thoughts are spiraling and you're feeling more distressed, maybe it's time to take a mental step back. Small pauses, mindful breaks, and even just breathing deeply can bring a lot of benefit. When you give your brain room to breathe, it's easier to see things for what they really are, instead of feeling like you're stuck in an endless traffic jam of your thoughts.

By understanding the mechanics of overthinking and its toll on your whole being, getting that control back isn't just a nice-to-have; it's crucial. It's about grounding yourself back in **reality** and letting those negative loops die out—giving your mind and body the rest it truly deserves.

In the end, mastering the art of letting go starts with spotting that overthinking and knowing when it's hijacking your peace. That fresh breath, that lighter step, it's all within arm's reach once you simply let yourself stop—for a moment—and start recognizing the patterns.

So, why not give it a try?

In Conclusion

In this chapter, you've taken a deep **dive** into understanding how to let go of the past and the **psychology** behind it. By releasing emotional **baggage** and stopping overthinking, your life can become more peaceful and fulfilling. You've learned about the ways your brain holds onto past experiences and the steps you can take to break free. Here's what stood out the most:

You've seen how your brain can cling to past experiences and how this can impact your feelings and life. The concept of **neuroplasticity** shows that your brain can change and help you let go of old patterns. There are psychological **benefits** such as reduced anxiety and improved emotional balance when you let go. Understanding attachment patterns is key to emotional **freedom**. It's important to recognize the difference between healthy reflection and harmful overthinking and **rumination**.

By grasping these key points, you're now **equipped** to start letting go of things that weigh you down and to embrace a life with more emotional freedom. Putting these ideas into action will not only improve your well-being but also help you handle future challenges with a clearer and more positive mindset. Go forth and start making these changes today!

Chapter 2: The Foundations of Emotional Healing

Have you ever wondered why some days you just can't shake that **bad feeling**? Or why certain **memories** seem to haunt you, no matter how hard you try to push them away? I know I have. This chapter is all about those moments and what you can do about them.

Picture yourself learning things that will help you make sense of all that **noise** in your head. You're about to unlock a version of yourself that's not held back by nagging feelings or past baggage. You'll dive into how **understanding** emotions and being aware of them can be a real game-changer. It's about taking those lingering unresolved feelings and finally facing them head-on.

Then there's the part where we talk about **resilience**. And no, it's not some far-off dream—it's something you can start building today. Feeling down? Yep, **self-compassion** can lift you up.

Ever wonder how your mind and **body** are connected? Trust me, this part's surprisingly interesting. The two are more linked than you might think.

I hope to light that spark of **curiosity** within you. This chapter won't just teach you—it'll lead you to a better understanding of yourself. Ready?

Emotional Intelligence and Self-Awareness

Let's chat about something super important - **emotional intelligence**. It's not just for people in therapy or self-help junkies. You can benefit from it, especially when dealing with emotional pain. Emotional intelligence has a few main parts, and getting good at them can really help on your path to healing.

First up, there's **self-awareness**. Basically, it means knowing what you're feeling and why you're feeling it. Sounds simple, right? But it can actually be kinda tricky. Being more self-aware means paying attention to your thoughts and emotions. Try to notice your reactions to things, sort of like being your own detective. Ask yourself questions like, "Why does this make me so mad?" or "Why do I feel sad about this?" It's about digging into your feelings without getting stuck in them.

Next is **self-regulation**. Picture a car with a good set of brakes. When things get heated, you can put the brakes on your emotional reactions. Self-regulation isn't about bottling up feelings, though. It's more about managing how and when they come out. Ever flipped out on someone then felt kinda dumb about it later? Self-regulation helps you keep those impulsive outbursts in check. Try counting to ten when you're stressed or imagine taking a big, calming breath.

There's also **empathy**, which is all about understanding how others feel. This can honestly do wonders for your own emotional healing. When you tap into someone else's feelings, it reminds you that you're not alone. Plus, helping others manage their feelings can make your own struggles feel less overwhelming.

Then we have **social skills**. Good ones aren't just for making friends or getting a promotion at work. They're about connecting with others on a deeper level, which can be really healing. Sharing experiences and talking things out with a friend can make emotional wounds feel less raw. It's like, "Hey, maybe I can survive this after all."

Finally, there's **motivation**. This one's about finding the drive to face and work through your emotions. It's the little push you need to get out of bed on rough days, even if it's just to take a walk or journal a bit.

So, how do you get more self-aware? Start with small steps. Journaling's a good way to kick things off. Jot down what happened during your day and how it made you feel. Check in with yourself during the day. Are you tense? Relaxed? Frustrated? Knowing this gives you a leg up on handling emotional pain, same as having a map when you're lost. Also, don't shy away from seeking feedback from trusted friends. Sometimes you miss stuff about yourself, and an outside perspective can be super helpful.

When you're self-aware, it really helps you to notice those emotional potholes before you trip into them. Feeling angry? Maybe it's not just about the overcooked dinner but about something way deeper. Catching these emotions early means you can address them before they snowball.

So how does all this help with complex feelings? Like we mentioned, life's full of twists and turns and different shades of gray. Sometimes you feel a lot of things all at once. Emotional intelligence can help sort out that tangled mess. Instead of feeling swamped by sadness, stress, and anger all at the same time, you start picking them apart.

Think of it like untangling earbuds: not fun, but totally necessary. Knowing which string goes where clears things up. You go from "I'm a crappy friend because I forgot her birthday" to "Actually, I'm overwhelmed at work, need more sleep, and should apologize." Suddenly, it feels more doable.

Remember, we aren't looking for perfect here, just progress. Notice your feelings, gently sort them out, and keep trying to adjust. Each step in emotional intelligence is a stride towards healing. Keep working at it, you'll find it's worth it. And hey, never underrate small victories. They're the ones that build up into your bigger healing moments.

The Impact of Unresolved Experiences

Unresolved emotional stuff can really mess with your mind and **body** over time. You've probably felt it yourself. Maybe something bad happened years ago, and you thought you'd moved on—only to have it pop up again out of nowhere. That's emotional **memory** for you. It's like, while your brain was busy storing all the good stuff, it also kept a special little file of everything awful that's ever happened to you. This file tends to open at the worst possible moments.

Emotional memory is tricky like that. While regular memories might fade or get fuzzy, emotional ones stick around with all their bad vibes intact. They're not just sitting there quietly, mind you. They're simmering, always ready to bubble up when triggered by something even slightly similar to the original event. It's like old wounds that won't fully heal. Remember how falling off a bike and scraping your knee at ten may have kept you off bikes for a while? Now amplify that when talking deep hurt like, say, betrayal or loss.

Ignoring these emotional wounds won't do any good. They don't just stay in your head; they like to jump into your **body** too. Ever notice how stressed-out folks always seem to have stomach trouble or constant headaches? That's emotional junk messing with their physical health. Yes, **stress** from unresolved experiences can show up as chronic tension, high blood pressure, or even ulcer risk. So, it's like carrying a heavy backpack every day—it wears you down over time.

Long-term, the real danger here is emotional wounds that you don't deal with. Think of them as landmines scattered across the landscape of your mind. Untriggered, they can make your life a sort of dangerous place to navigate. PTSD, **anxiety**, depression—they're not just buzzwords. Left unchecked, those old hurts will take a serious toll on your mental **health**.

When it goes on long enough, you might start avoiding situations that could trigger those unresolved feelings. So, you isolate yourself, stop doing stuff you love, or push people away. And that can lead to even more emotional wreckage. Also, **relationships** take a major hit. It's tough to be open and genuine with others when you're on guard all the time.

Your performance at work or school could dive too. Hard to stay focused when your mind is dealing with old pain. Your sleep quality could tank, making it a struggle just to get through the day. Gauge the energy drain that comes from carrying these unresolved bits and bobs around between perceived vulnerability or slipping in performance. Like potholes on a busy street—they fast become hazards you don't anticipate.

This stuff really makes life tough. So what can you do about it? Face them — you know, those unresolved experiences. Work on them, instead of tucking them away. Deal with what's hurting you, no matter how nasty it might seem. You don't have to figure this out by yourself. Find someone who gets it—a friend or even a professional like a **therapist**. Taking that step might just change things around significantly.

Dealing with your emotional baggage isn't easy. It's essential. It means better health, both in your mind and your body. Plus, you'd likely have a more peaceful and fulfilling life. Less stress, better relationships, more joy—not something you'd pass up on, right?

Ignoring those old wounds just won't cut it. Time to face them, heal, and move forward. So, are you ready to start the **healing** process?

Building Resilience Through Self-Compassion

Let's get comfy and chat about **self-compassion**. It might sound like a fancy concept, but trust me, it's pretty simple and incredibly useful.

So, what's self-compassion all about? In a nutshell, it means treating yourself with the same kindness and understanding you'd offer a close friend. Weird, right? We're usually our own worst critics. But this self-compassion thing can actually help you **bounce back** emotionally. By being kind to yourself, you create a safety net. Life's rollercoaster doesn't feel as scary because you know you've got your own back.

Self-compassion breaks down into three parts: being kind to yourself, realizing you're not alone, and staying aware of the present moment.

Being kind to yourself means ditching that inner voice that's always putting you down. Imagine telling yourself supportive words, just like you would to a bestie. For example, you could say, "You messed up, but it's okay. You're only human." See how that changes things? This gentle approach pulls you away from self-criticism. You stop beating yourself up. With practice, being gentle with yourself becomes your go-to when you're facing tough times. And when you're kinder to yourself, **emotional healing** isn't such an uphill battle. You grow. You learn. You bounce back faster.

Now for another slice: realizing you're not alone. Feeling isolated is common when you're going through rough patches. Here's where self-compassion swoops in. By acknowledging that others through similar struggles, you lessen that sense of loneliness. It's like joining an invisible but global support group. Whenever life throws you curveballs, remind yourself that you're in good company. Others have faced similar woes and survived, even thrived. This thought itself is comforting. It provides a sense of interconnected **resilience**, which softens life's blows.

Onto the last part: staying aware of the present moment. **Mindfulness** is all about being right here, right now—without getting dragged into past regrets or future worries. Practicing this helps you see things as they are, not as you fear they might become. This way, you stop blowing problems out of proportion, creating space for calmer, more measured responses to what's happening. Imagine taking a few deep breaths and realizing that, in this moment, you're okay. Problems might still be there, but your mind feels clearer without that overthinking fog.

Combining these three aspects, self-compassion turns into your emotional toolkit. Let's face it. Life's challenges aren't going anywhere. But with self-compassion, you bounce back quicker, heal deeper, and grow stronger. You become your own best ally, a force to be reckoned with.

And hey, treating yourself kindly isn't just for kicks. It's essential for **self-growth**. You're constantly evolving—at your own pace and in your own way. Every time you practice self-compassion, you give yourself the fertile ground you need to grow. The world becomes a friendlier place, and you **recover** from setbacks with more ease.

Isn't that something worth striving for?

The Connection Between Mind and Body

You might not always think about it, but your **mind** and **body** are like best friends—they're constantly chatting. When it comes to **emotional** healing, this connection is super important.

Ever notice how stress can give you a headache, make your shoulders tense up, or even mess with your stomach? That's your body's way of saying, "Hey, something's not right!" Over time, stress can wreak havoc on your sleep, weaken your **immune** system, and even jack up your blood pressure. It's crazy how much a bad mood can impact your physical health, right?

When you're dealing with emotional wounds or overthinking the past, it's not just in your head. It affects your whole body. Your muscles stay tight, you might feel **exhausted** all the time, and sometimes it's even hard to focus. It's like lugging around a heavy backpack that's constantly weighing you down.

Your physical health has just as much power to mess with your emotions. Ever had a nasty cold and felt super irritable or down? Or how about after a killer workout, feeling on top of the world? That's because your physical state has a huge influence on your emotional well-being. Eating well and getting enough sleep aren't just fancy health tips; they're the building blocks of feeling good.

But **healing** isn't a solo gig. It's like a two-way street—fixing your mind helps your body, and taking care of your body heals your mind, too. Working on emotional health through stuff like **mindfulness**, talking it out with friends, or even seeking professional help can lead to better sleep, less muscle tension, and lower stress hormones in your body.

When you take care of your body, you're also giving your mind a boost. Exercise releases endorphins—those awesome chemicals that make you feel happy. Plus, a balanced diet gives your brain the nutrients it needs to keep chugging along. Just stepping outside for some fresh air can make a world of difference.

In my opinion, this link between mind and body is pure magic. It's an endless cycle that's always spinning. Get control of one part, and the other one improves too—it's a win-win. And don't underestimate the power of simple things in life, like strolling through a park, chatting with a friend, or just sitting quietly. All this creates space for both your mind and body to catch a breather and heal.

So next time you're having a rough day or feeling low, try something different. Take a moment to focus on your breath, stretch out, or even get moving a bit. Small steps can lead to big shifts, freeing you bit by bit from the past. You'll feel lighter, both in your head and in your body.

When you work on syncing your mind and body, you're playing the long game of living stress-free and emotionally sound. This isn't just feel-good talk; it's practical stuff anyone can get on board with. So, live a bit, stretch a bit, care a lot. It's really the combo of mind and body that sets you free.

Back and forth, weave and bob—two partners in this grand seesaw act of life. You get to navigate this daily—that powerful link between your mind and body. So go easy on both. They're your lifelong team.

In Conclusion

In this chapter, you've **explored** some foundational aspects of emotional healing, which can be super important for personal **growth**. By wrapping your head around these ideas better, you can take active steps towards a healthier, more balanced life. Here's what we've covered:

Emotional **intelligence** helps you understand and manage your feelings better, which is crucial for healing. Being **self-aware** allows you to recognize when you're emotionally hurt and take steps to address it. Unresolved emotional experiences can mess with your mental and physical health if you don't properly deal with them. Practicing **self-compassion** can make you more resilient and help in the healing process. There's a strong **connection** between your mental state and physical well-being; taking care of one helps improve the other.

By putting what you've learned into practice, you can start making meaningful **changes** in your life. Remember, it's all about small steps toward understanding yourself better and caring for your emotional and physical health. You've got the **power** to heal and grow. So go ahead, kick-start this positive change today!

Chapter 3: The Dichotomy of Control

Ever wondered why some people seem so **relaxed**, even when everything's going wrong? It's like life's **chaos** doesn't bother them one bit. In this chapter, we're gonna crack that mystery together.

You know, life throws so much at you—some of it bad, some good. It's easy to feel **overwhelmed**, right? But here's the twist – not everything is yours to **control**. Now, that might seem like a downer at first. But, on digging deeper, it's really kinda freeing. You'll see why soon enough.

Imagine your **energy** is like a limited battery. You'd want to use that battery wisely, wouldn't you? By figuring out what's in your control and what's not, you can save that precious energy for the stuff that actually matters. You're gonna learn how to do this, using some straight-talk and practical steps.

You'll start by sorting what's controllable from what's not, like separating apples from oranges. Then, it's all about making **peace** with the uncontrollable stuff. Yeah, it's easier said than done, but totally doable. And once you master that, you'll be a pro at focusing your energy where it counts.

Ready to get started? Trust me, this chapter will **change** the way you see things. Let's dive in and shake up your **perspective** on life's challenges!

Distinguishing Between Controllable and Uncontrollable Factors

Let's dive into the nitty-gritty of **control**—what you can manage and what's out of your hands. The Stoics had this idea, and it's surprisingly relevant today. Basically, they put stuff into two buckets: things you can control and stuff you just can't. It might sound like common sense, but let's dig deeper.

What goes into the "I can control this" bucket? It's stuff like your **actions**, your **thoughts**, and your reactions to things. Yep, all internal stuff. You get to decide how you respond to life's kicks and curves. On the flip side, things like the weather, other people's actions, or even your past are beyond your control. You didn't write the script to your life's soap opera, but you've got a say in your own lines.

Why does this matter today? Because let's face it, getting hung up on things outside your control is exhausting. Think of it as a GPS for your attention and effort. If you're spending hours dwelling on why Jane at work didn't give you credit for that project, you're burning brain fuel on something you can't control. But if you focus on giving your best for the next project, the energy's directed to a meaningful outcome. Makes sense, right?

Now, let's talk perks—what you gain by focusing on what you can actually control. For starters, it's a **stress-buster**. When you let go of stuff over which you have no control, there's a kind of mental relaxation. Your mind gets room to breathe. It's also good for your **confidence**. Focusing on actions within your control gives you a sense of achievement, which compounds over time as you meet small goals one after another.

And let's not forget, it's pretty empowering. You don't wait on others to decide your worth or success. You get to create it. When you're in the driver's seat of your own decisions and reactions, there's a profound satisfaction in knowing you've got a handle on at least part of the chaos life throws at you.

But here's the hump we all need to get over—common myths about control that mess with our emotions. One big myth is thinking that with enough effort, you can control everything. Bad news: life's like a box of chocolates, full of surprises and beyond your mastery. Holding onto this myth can end up messing with your anxiety levels. You keep thinking, "If only I did/made/fixed this, everything would be perfect!" Spoiler alert: perfection's a pipe dream.

Another more subtle myth is that relinquishing control equals failure. You might think that if you admit you can't manage everything, it's like giving up. But acknowledging your limits isn't defeat—it's **wisdom**. It's understanding where to channel your effort for maximum impact.

Plus, control-freak tendencies can screw with **relationships**, too. Pinning expectations or actions on those around you based on what you think you can sway ends up in frustration—for both you and them. Trust me, hinting your partner into getting you flowers doesn't wield the same magic as when it's their idea.

So, next time you find yourself tangled, remember these Stoic notions. Sort out what you can genuinely influence and what you can't. With practice, you'll start seeing the impact on your mental state and overall **happiness**. It's like packing light for a Rocky mountain hike; feeling lighter and definitely more prepared for the trek. Prioritizing what truly requires your efforts can flip the script on how you deal with life.

It's like the old saying goes, "Grant me the serenity to accept the things I cannot change, courage to change the things I can, and wisdom to know the difference." You're just picking up bits of **wisdom** as you go. And those bits? They're gold.

Accepting What Cannot Be Changed

You know that feeling when you finally let go of something that's been **bugging** you forever? It's like your mind does a little shift, making room for peace. See, your brain loves to hold onto things – what someone said years ago, decisions you regret, all that jazz. But when you tell your brain it's okay to let those things be, it's like cleaning out a cluttered attic. You can breathe easier. You walk around feeling lighter. And suddenly, the chains of old worries don't pull you back anymore. That feeling? It's **emotional freedom**.

Makes you wonder, right? Like, what if letting go isn't the same as giving up? It's like when you're climbing a hill. Accepting means saying, "Okay, that patch of rocks is rough. Let me step around it." Giving up is just sitting down and saying you'll never make it to the top. **Acceptance** is an active choice. It's powerful. It's seeing things as they are, not as you wish they'd be.

But let's not mix things up – accepting doesn't mean you're throwing in the towel. Nah. It's about recognizing what you can't control (the past, how others act, or random life events) and what you can control (how you react to those things).

This process, this whole acceptance gig we're talking about, it's like your GPS recalculating when you miss a turn. You don't just stop and wait on the side of the road. You find another way forward. And with it comes this sweet bonus – less **emotional pain**.

Think about it. Every time you wrestle with what-ifs or could've-beens, you're exhausting your emotional reserves. That regret or anger or bitterness? It's eating away at you. But when you go,

"Okay, that's done. What's next?" you're saving a world of emotional energy. Think of acceptance as an emotional ointment. It soothes. It heals. You don't get stuck in the same loop of pain.

Feels **contradictory** sometimes, doesn't it? Like, aren't you sorta conditioned to be a go-getter, always seeking change? It's a mindset shift. Accepting things you can't change doesn't mean you stop aiming higher or wanting things to be better. It's more about being realistic. Don't beat yourself up for things that are beyond your control.

When you look at those uncontrollable parts and say, "I'm cool with this," you're actually reclaiming power. It's different from defeat. It's choosing inner **peace** over constant struggle.

But always remember this bit: the aim isn't perfection. It's about making gradual **progress**. Today you might only manage to release a slight grudge. Tomorrow, maybe you let go of something bigger.

Alright, enough talk. It's time to practice. Next time an old hurt pops up – stop, take a breath, tell yourself it's okay, and let it drift away. You're not giving up. You're giving yourself **permission** to move on. And in doing so, you're a step closer to that emotional freedom we all crave.

Now, get out there and feel the difference acceptance makes. You'll thank yourself later.

Focusing Energy on Actionable Areas

Let's talk about the idea of locus of control. It's a fancy-sounding term, but in simple terms, it's all about what you believe you can **control** in your life. Think of it as two zones: stuff you can do something about and stuff you just can't. People with a strong internal locus of control believe they have the power to shape their own destiny. They see themselves more in the driver's seat. On the flip side, those with an external locus of control think outside forces, like luck or other people, hold the reins. Not surprisingly, having an internal locus is way more empowering.

Every day, you're faced with things you can control and things you can't. The trick is to figure out which is which. It's like sorting laundry. You don't want to waste time ironing out wrinkles in socks when what you need is to press your dress shirt for tomorrow's big meeting. Similarly, put your **energy** into areas where you can actually make a difference.

Here's how to figure out and prioritize the areas in your life where you can take **action**:

• Identify your issues: Make a list. Seriously, just write down the things that bug you.

• Sort your list: Decide which of these you can influence and which you can't. Can't control the weather? Put that in the "no-go" pile. Can control how prepared you are for a rainy day? That goes in the "action" pile.

• Prioritize: Not everything in the "action" pile is equally urgent. What needs your attention most? Deal with that first.

Putting effort into things you can control isn't just about getting stuff done. There's a huge mental **benefit** that comes with it. Get a grip on what you can manage, and guess what? You start feeling more competent. You're less likely to wallow in self-pity or feel overwhelmed. It's like your brain gets a little high-five every time you tackle something successfully.

When you focus on things outside your control, it can really mess with your head. You end up stressed, frustrated, and anxious. It's almost like trying to win a game where the rules keep changing. And who likes playing games where you can't win? So why put yourself through that?

On the other hand, when you put your energy into things you can control, you gain **confidence** and reduce anxiety. It's empowering. It gives you a sense of **purpose**. Tackling manageable problems kind of snowballs into bigger successes. Basically, it's a win-win.

So there you have it. Start by shifting your **focus** onto where you can truly make a difference. Target those areas, and you'll find more clarity, control, and peace in your life. You're no longer just a passive observer but an active participant in your own life. It's like moving from the audience to center stage. Ready to take charge? Go sort that laundry – err, life. You'll feel better for it.

Developing a Proactive Mindset

A proactive **mindset** makes a world of difference. Imagine feeling like you're steering your own ship instead of just bobbing along with the waves. That's what being proactive is all about. When you're proactive, you **think** ahead and take steps to influence your own life's direction. This lets you feel a lot more in control.

So, how do you go from just reacting to things—and freaking out a bit when they don't go as planned—to actually taking **charge**? It starts with small shifts in your mind. Start by noticing which problems in your life you can do something about, and which you can't. Don't waste time stressing over the stuff you can't control. Instead, put your **energy** into the things you can change.

Think of it this way: when you're reacting, you're like a leaf getting tossed around by the wind. You're just responding to whatever comes your way. But when you take charge, you become more like the tree—standing firm and influencing the direction, making **decisions** that impact your life in bigger ways than you may realize.

One way to do this is by setting specific, doable **goals**. Don't make grand plans that are hard to achieve. Instead, set smaller, more achievable targets. This includes asking questions like, "What do I want to accomplish today?" or "What steps can I take to solve this problem?"

Switching your mindset from reactive to proactive might take some time. But, like any habit or new skill, the more you work at it, the better you get. Start with baby steps—make one proactive decision each day. Over time, these small **actions** add up and make a massive impact on your life. You begin to notice you're approaching problems differently, not as scary monsters but as challenges you can face head-on.

Now, let's dig into the perks of having a proactive mindset over the long term. It's not just about today or tomorrow—it's about your whole life changing in little but important ways. First, your stress levels drop. Think about it: when you're in control, you don't get thrown off balance by every little hiccup. You handle things better because you've already thought ahead. This sense of control also boosts your confidence. Knowing you can face challenges head-on gives you a huge mental win. Let's not forget the added bonus of feeling optimistic. When you believe you have the power to change stuff in your life, you automatically start seeing things in a brighter light.

There's also personal **growth**. A proactive mindset makes you more resilient. Every time you choose to take action, you build a kind of mental muscle. When you face difficulties, instead of feeling defeated, you feel more equipped and less phased.

In conclusion, switching to a proactive mindset isn't just a quick fix. It's the start of a lifelong habit that improves your well-being, personal growth, and overall happiness. It sets you up for a brighter and more fulfilling future. So why not start now? Take control of your life and see how much better things can be.

Practical Exercise: Applying the Dichotomy of Control

Alright, let's dive right in. Picture a **tough situation** you're facing right now. Got it? Great. This exercise will help you break it down, make sense of it, and lighten your load a bit.

First, think about that challenging situation. Maybe you're struggling with a project at work, family drama, or trying to patch up a relationship. Just pick one thing that's **weighing** you down the most.

Now, jot down all the parts of the situation. Don't hold back – write down everything that's stressing you out, every little detail.

Take a breather and **sort** those parts into things you can control and things you can't. It might seem obvious, but sometimes it's tricky to separate the two. Ask yourself: Do you have a say in this part? If you do, it goes under "can control." If not, toss it into "can't control."

For the things you can **control**, it's time to take action. Write down some concrete steps to tackle those. If something's up to you, try breaking it into smaller, manageable tasks. Say you're behind on a project – why not block out some time in your calendar to get a head start? Come up with specific, doable tasks that bring you closer to a solution.

Here's the kicker for the stuff you can't control – let it go. Easier said than done, I know. But **acknowledging** you can't change something can be freeing. Give yourself permission not to waste energy on what's unchangeable. It's tough but necessary. Focus on acceptance and move on.

Feel different? This exercise should **shift** your perspective a bit. Notice how focusing on actionable stuff makes you feel more in control and less stressed. No need for that extra weight of impossible demands, right?

Don't stop here. Make this a **habit**. Every new tough situation? Go through these steps again. Over time, this process becomes second nature. You'll start recognizing what's within your reach and what's not from the get-go.

The idea here is pretty simple, yet it's super **powerful**. Once you focus on what you can change, you spend less time worrying about things outside your control. You'll find a massive weight lifts off your shoulders when you let go of trying to manage the unmanageable. That's a recipe for peace.

I promise, it gets easier with practice. Treat it like a muscle you're working on. Keep at it. You'll start noticing the difference it makes in how you handle life's ups and downs.

Simple, isn't it? Go ahead, give it your best shot. It's about making life a little easier, one "letting go" moment at a time.

In Conclusion

You've **delved** into the art of distinguishing between what's within your **control** and what isn't, and how this can seriously boost your emotional well-being. Putting these ideas into practice can help you live a more **fulfilling** and less stressful life by zeroing in on what you can actually **influence**.

The Stoic concept of the dichotomy of control isn't just ancient wisdom; it's a **practical** guide for modern living. By focusing on factors you can control, you're setting yourself up for success and peace of mind. It's easy to get caught up in common **myths** about control, but recognizing these can be a game-changer for your emotions.

Remember, **acceptance** isn't throwing in the towel; it's about being emotionally flexible. Adopting a **proactive** mindset can lead to some serious personal growth. You've got the power to make a real difference in your life by prioritizing what you can change and making peace with what you can't.

So, why not give it a shot? Focus on what truly matters, and you might just find yourself living a life that's more in tune with your values and goals. It's all about taking those small steps towards a bigger, better picture of your life.

Chapter 4: Mastering Nonjudgmental Awareness

Ever had that split second where your **mind** wanders, and you start judging yourself or others? Well, I have. In this chapter, we're going to explore something different—nonjudgmental **awareness**. It'll open things up in ways you've never thought possible.

Imagine if you could **observe** your thoughts without getting all tangled up in them. You're not reacting or attaching any feelings—just noticing. Sounds pretty freeing, right? This chapter will help you do just that. You'll learn how to watch those thoughts float by, like clouds in the sky. No fuss, no stress—kinda cool, huh?

Have you ever felt overwhelmed by your **feelings**? Like, one minute you're okay, and then—bam—stress hits hard. You can change that. You'll see how staying **objective** can actually chill things out. Plus, there's a bit on how you can better manage those rollercoaster **emotions**.

Here's a little bonus—want to really nail down this nonjudgmental stuff? I've included a practical **exercise**, something you can practice to get better at observing without all that mental noise. It's like a mini reset for your mind. Let's embark on this fascinating **path**, and who knows what levels of peace you might reach?

The Essence of Nonjudgmental Thinking

Let's dive into what nonjudgmental **awareness** is all about and why it matters. Nonjudgmental thinking stems from **mindfulness** practices. It's like noticing your thoughts, feelings, or surroundings without slapping labels like "good" or "bad" on them. You just see things as they are. Picture yourself sitting beside a stream, watching the water flow without trying to change its course—that's how you want to approach your own mind.

Why's this important? Well, it can give your **mental** health a real boost. You know how your mind can sometimes be like that annoying neighbor who never stops complaining? Everything has to meet their sky-high standards. But what if you could tune out that negativity? By not judging your thoughts, you dial down your stress and anxiety. It's like turning down the volume on harsh self-talk and cranking up the peace. Simple as that.

Let's break it down further with a cool technique called "**RAIN**." It's super helpful for developing nonjudgmental awareness. You'll love it.

First, Recognize: Just notice what's happening. It's like saying, "Hey there, thought" without getting all worked up. Imagine you're in the middle of a hectic day, and suddenly you feel really tense. You recognize that feeling. "Oh, I'm feeling super tense right now."

Next, Allow: Let whatever it is just be. Don't try to fix it or push it away. Just sit with it. Going back to that tension—you just let it hang out. It's okay to feel this way. Instead of thinking you should "snap out of it," you give yourself permission to feel whatever bubbles up. Pretty liberating, right?

Then, Investigate: Get curious. Ask yourself why you're feeling that way, but don't judge it. This isn't the Spanish Inquisition; it's more like Sherlock Holmes, you know? What's behind that tension? Did something trigger it? Maybe a deadline's looming, or someone said something that rubbed you the wrong way. Poke around a bit to see what's lurking underneath.

Finally, Non-identify: This is a game-changer. Realize that you're not your thoughts or **emotions**. They're just passing clouds in the sky of your mind. You don't need to act on them—you can just let them float by. It's such a relief to know that a moment of anger doesn't define you or make you an angry person. You're so much bigger than that.

The beauty of "RAIN" is that it helps you come to terms with things instead of running away or getting stuck in a loop of overthinking. Think of it like giving your mind a relaxing bath instead of letting it marinate in worries and judgments.

In the long run, mastering nonjudgmental thinking can change how you see the world and yourself. It leads to lower **stress** and greater emotional health. You'll start noticing you're not as reactive as you used to be. The stressors might still be there, but they don't have that same grip on you. It's kind of like having an umbrella in the rain—things might be wet around you, but you're not getting soaked.

There you have it! Nonjudgmental thinking isn't about becoming a monk or living in isolation. It's a practical **tool** to make peace with your messiest thoughts and emotions. When you're able to step back and say, "This, too, shall pass," life gets a lot simpler. I think we all need a bit of that right now. Don't you?

Observing Thoughts Without Attachment

You know how your **thoughts** sometimes keep spinning around in your head, making everything seem all big and messy? Well, one way to calm things down is by giving yourself a bit of mental space. Imagine treating your thoughts like they're not solid truths but just passing events. Kinda like **clouds** in the sky. They come, they go, and you don't have to grab onto any of them.

This idea is a big deal because, often, you treat your thoughts as if they're the absolute truth. Thoughts like, "I'm not good enough" or "I always screw up," can really sting and hang around in your mind. But guess what? They're not facts. They're just thoughts. If you can start seeing them that way, they lose a lot of their power. This is where the concept of **cognitive defusion** comes in.

Ever heard of cognitive defusion? It's all about creating some distance between you and your thoughts. Typically, when a bad thought pops up, you grab onto it quickly, and it affects how you feel and behave. Defusion teaches you to see these thoughts without getting hooked on them. Think of it like watching a scary movie. When you remember it's just a movie, it loses its scare factor, right? That's cognitive defusion at work.

A neat trick to practice this is using the "Leaves on a Stream" **visualization** technique. It's super simple and kinda fun, too. Here's how it works:

Close your eyes and take a deep breath. Picture yourself sitting next to a stream on a comfy, warm day. Imagine putting each of your thoughts on a leaf and gently setting it on the water. Just watch it float away.

Let's say a thought pops up like, "I messed up at work yesterday." Place that thought on a leaf and just watch it drift down the stream. Don't chase it, don't jump in after it—just let it go. Picture another thought about a conversation you regret. Put that on a leaf as well and let it float away.

What's cool about this **practice** is you're not trying to stop your thoughts or change them. You're just observing them. Kinda like a play. You're in the audience, not on the stage. This way, thoughts start to feel less threatening, and you see them as just thoughts, not who you are.

But sometimes, it's tricky to remember to practice these techniques, especially when you're caught up in the middle of a thought storm. One way to make it easier is by setting small reminders throughout the day. Like, a sticky note on your mirror saying, "Thoughts aren't facts." It gives you a gentle nudge to step back and practice nonjudgmental **awareness**.

In my opinion, this approach was a game-changer for me. Instead of getting stuck in a web of my thinking, I started feeling freer. It's kinda like when you've been carrying around a heavy backpack all day, and you finally take it off. Feels lighter, doesn't it?

So, think of these skills as your tools for carving out that mental space. Practice them a bit daily, and eventually, they just become a part of how you think. Baby steps go a long way. It's about allowing yourself to notice your thoughts without holding onto them.

When you get the hang of observing without **attachment**, it's like you're building inner peace. You'll see thoughts come and go, and you won't be dragged along for the ride. It's like standing in the middle of a busy street but feeling calm and still. It's **freedom** from the mental chaos.

Reducing Stress Through Objectivity

It's super helpful to look at things from a more **objective** point of view. When you do that, you're less likely to react emotionally, and your stress can drop. Why? Because instead of being all caught up in how things feel, you're seeing them for what they actually are.

Think about when someone cuts you off in traffic. Yeah, it's annoying, but if you start thinking they did it on purpose, you get mad, your heart rate goes up, and **stress** levels shoot through the roof. But what if you look at it like maybe they just didn't see you, or they're distracted because they're having a bad day? Suddenly, it's less personal. You can shrug it off easier. Just like that, poof, less stress.

What if you decide to rethink annoying **situations**? When you see things from different angles, you're not just stuck seeing it as bad. This can keep you stable emotionally. Say your friend cancels your meetup. Instead of thinking they don't care, what if they're genuinely swamped with work? Seeing things in a new light often reveals there's more to the story. Your emotions won't control you, and you'll feel more balanced.

Wanna try something that helps for real? It's called "**Describe**, Don't Judge." The idea is, when a situation stirs up emotions, just describe it without getting all judgy. Let's practice.

Imagine you've got a huge work **presentation**. Your instinct might be to think, "Ugh, I'm gonna mess this up, I always screw things up!" Instead, describe what's happening. Like, "I have a presentation at work. I'm feeling nervous." That's it. No judgment, just facts. Try it for a week and notice how saying just what it is can lighten the emotional load.

Another angle – think about this: you're late for an important meeting. The normal rush of panic hits. Instead of thinking, "I'm so terrible, how could I let this happen!" try saying, "I left home later than I wanted, and now I'm running late." This simple shift in **perspective** stops the stress spiral and helps you focus on just fixing the problem.

It won't always be easy. Those pesky judgments creep up. Get too busy thinking about who's to blame or why things always seem to go wrong, and you'll miss the chance to lessen stress. It's kind of freeing to see things just as they are.

This technique's pretty useful for **emotions** too. Got a situation making you feel low? Describe it. "I had a conversation with a friend that left me feeling kinda down." Not, "They're always making me feel awful." Notice the shift? One's loaded with judgment and assumptions, the other's clear and factual. Less emotional charge, less stress.

Sound too simple? Give it some time. Working on being just factual rather than judgmental can help train your brain to calm down more often. It's like teaching yourself to chill. **Objectivity** isn't about being cold or unfeeling, it's about seeing things clearly.

So next time that stressful event pops up, remember – describe, don't judge. It can be a game-changer in learning how to keep your cool. Sure, it takes practice, like any new skill, but the payoff is worth it. Less stress, more calm, and a better way to handle life's little hiccups. Trust me, looking at things this way can make a big difference, and you deserve that peace.

Enhancing Emotional Regulation

Let's talk about how being aware without judging can actually make you better at handling and responding to your **emotions**. It feels kinda like you're turning off a constant background analysis that usually goes on without you noticing. You're just *there*, experiencing things as they happen. Imagine being able to feel sad without thinking, "I'm so weak" or happy without worrying about what's coming next. It's **liberating**, really.

By practicing this, you start recognizing that feelings are just feelings. Like clouds passing by on a windy day, they come and go if you let them. You don't have to chase after them or push them away. They're just there to be noticed...not ruled by. When you simply notice your emotions, you're more likely to **respond** in a way that's calm and balanced rather than reactive or defensive. This makes a huge difference in how you handle everything from minor annoyances to big life challenges.

Now, let's dive into **emotional granularity**. It's a fancy term, but it's pretty simple. Emotional granularity means being able to identify and understand your feelings in detail. Instead of just being "sad" or "mad," you can pinpoint that you're "disappointed," "frustrated," or "anxious." This isn't just cool trivia; it actually helps you manage your emotions better.

Why's this so important? Well, if you know exactly what you're feeling, you can deal with it more effectively. It's like having a detailed map of your feelings. When you know you're "frustrated" instead of just "mad," you might realize that having a clearer plan or talking things out could help. If you're "disappointed," you might focus on adjusting your expectations. The more detailed your understanding, the better your **response**.

Here's a tip to really boost your emotional **awareness**: try the "Emotion Naming" technique. It's kinda like when you've got a cluttered closet and you finally start labeling things. When an emotion bubbles up, take a moment to name it. Is it anger, or is it irritation? Are you really just tired? Naming your feelings can make them less overwhelming. It creates a bit of distance, which makes it easier to think about what you can do next.

Try to set aside a bit of time each day—maybe during your wind-down at night—to reflect on the emotions you've felt. List them out if you need to. It might seem tedious at first but stick with it. This habit can really improve your ability to **manage** your emotions over time.

The more you practice naming your emotions, the more natural it becomes. Soon, you'll notice patterns in your feelings and how they influence your behavior. This awareness gives you the power to make different choices, ones that align more with how you actually want to live your life.

And through all of this, keep that mindset of nonjudgmental awareness. Look at your emotions as signals, not signs of failure or flaws. You're just a human, figuring stuff out like everyone else. Practice makes perfect—not perfection. Just **progress**. Feelings are complicated, but they're also pretty predictable once you get to know them.

That's the essence of mastering nonjudgmental awareness to enhance your emotional regulation. Identifying what you're feeling and responding without rushing to judge yourself can transform how you experience life's ups and downs. Keep it simple, stay curious, and your emotional world will start making a lot more sense.

Practical Exercise: Nonjudgmental Observation

Ready to dive into some hands-on action? Let's explore **nonjudgmental awareness** with a practical exercise. Get comfy and see where it takes you.

Find a quiet, cozy spot where you won't be interrupted. It could be your favorite chair or a snug corner of the room. The idea is to be somewhere you can just be without distractions. Mute your devices, close the door if you need to – this time is all about you.

Close your eyes and take a few deep **breaths** to calm down. Let yourself sink into that relaxed state. Feel your lungs fill up and release all that air slowly. It's like inviting calmness to wash over you. In and out, nice and easy.

Start noticing your **thoughts**, feelings, and body sensations without trying to change them. If a thought pops up about that embarrassing thing you did in high school, don't try to wrangle it away. Just let it be. Feeling a bit of tension in your back? Acknowledge it, but don't fuss over it. These are simply passing guests in your mind's living room.

As you watch, label each **experience** simply as "thought," "feeling," or "sensation" without adding more. You don't need to unravel why the thought about that high school mishap popped up. Just label it with, "thought." If you feel sad, slap a "feeling" label on it. Whatever is happening in your body – "sensation." It's like you're sorting socks, not writing an essay.

If you catch yourself judging, just notice it and go back to neutral watching. This is bound to happen. Maybe you're thinking, "Wow, that was dumb." Instead of spiraling, just nudge yourself back to labeling: "judgment" and then, boop – back to observing.

Keep doing this for 5-10 minutes, and try to do it for longer over time. Don't stress about the exact time. Set a timer if it helps. Just build this **habit** at your own pace. Maybe today is a five-minute session, and next week, you want to stretch it to ten. The key here is to create a regular practice that grows naturally.

After you're done, think about what you experienced and any **insights** you had. Sit for a moment and reflect. Were there a lot of thoughts? Strong feelings? Perhaps a sensation that stood out? Did you learn something about how your mind works? Jot down anything noteworthy. This isn't for assessment but for understanding yourself better.

It's kind of like observing a rush of people in a busy plaza – different faces, reactions, and movements. You're the calm **observer**, seeing it all without getting caught up. Keep at it, and see how this **exercise** opens up new pathways for you.

In Conclusion

This chapter has given you deeper **insights** into the importance of nonjudgmental awareness and how it boosts your mental well-being. Through the various **techniques** and exercises shared, it's clear that adopting an objective perspective towards your thoughts and feelings can significantly lower **stress** and improve emotional regulation. Let's sum up the essence of what you've learned.

You've explored the basics and importance of adopting nonjudgmental **awareness**, the steps in the "RAIN" technique to help practice it, and the idea of seeing thoughts as passing events to create mental distance. You've also been introduced to **visualization** techniques like "Leaves on a Stream" for thought observation, and practical exercises to observe thoughts without judgment and practice emotional **regulation**.

As you mull over this chapter, consider putting these techniques into practice in your daily life. The **skills** you gain here will empower you to manage thoughts and emotions more effectively, fostering a state of peace and balance. By weaving these habits into your routine, you'll further enhance your ability to experience each moment as it comes, free from unnecessary judgments. Keep applying these **concepts**—they're your tools for a better, more mindful life.

Chapter 5: The Art of Self-Distancing

Ever found yourself caught in an emotional **whirlwind**? You've been there, right? The more you try to keep your cool, the worse it gets. But what if there was a way to take a step back and see things clearly, even when your feelings are going haywire? In this chapter, we'll dive into the **technique** of distancing yourself from your emotions and gaining some much-needed perspective.

I'm convinced that mastering this skill can be a **game-changer** in how you tackle life's challenges. When you're not at the mercy of your emotions, you can view situations more objectively. You'll find yourself in a better position to **problem-solve** and think outside the box. And believe me, once you dial down that emotional intensity, things often don't seem as bad as you first thought.

Let's make this practical with some simple **exercises** tailored just for you. You'll learn how to momentarily step out of your usual mindset and see things from different angles. It might seem like magic, but it's really about **practice**. You'll feel a weight lift off your shoulders and discover solutions more quickly.

So, let's dive in... we've got some fascinating ground to cover. Get ready to add a **tool** to your arsenal that could make your life a whole lot easier – and who couldn't use that?

Now, flip the page, and let's embark on this journey to master the art of self-**distancing**. Trust me, you're in for an eye-opening experience!

Creating Psychological Space from Emotions

Psychological distance might sound a bit odd at first, but trust me, it's a **game-changer**. It's all about finding a gap between you and your thoughts or feelings. Not too far off—just a little space to breathe, giving your mind a break. When **emotions** hit hard, that break acts like a buffer. Instead of getting totally swamped, you step back and, suddenly, those wild feelings become more manageable and less intimidating.

Think about watching a wild movie. When you're in the thick of it, every twist and tear feels like it's happening to you. But then imagine hitting pause. You get a moment to process, to think, to breathe. Creating psychological distance does just that for your emotions. By mentally stepping back, you see the scene clearer, less charged. Those towering feelings become hills, not mountains.

Ever heard of stepping outside yourself? Not literally, though. It's handy, like turning into your own advisor or friend's friend. This is where the **"Third-Person Perspective"** trick comes into play. Here's the scoop: when things get overwhelming, address yourself by name. Like, instead of "Why am I feeling so nervous?" say "Why is [your name] feeling so nervous?"

Here's how it helps out:

• **Calm The Storm**: Addressing yourself by name creates that buffer. Emotions cool off a bit. It's like looking at a problem someone else is having, and we all know things often look simpler from the outside.

• **Clearer View**: Distance yourself from strong feelings, and you'll see solutions or perspectives you might miss otherwise. Think of it as gaining a new lens—a much clearer one.

• **Rationality Rules**: Dampen the heat of emotions, and you make decisions with your cooler, more rational mind. Panic and anxiety have less power over you.

Imagine a heated **argument** with a close friend. Emotions flare up, words get thrown around. But step away for a moment... what happens? Chances are, if you talk to yourself in the third person, "Why is [your name] so worked up?" you might realize the issue isn't that massive. Maybe it's simple miscommunication, one a calmer you can address.

Create snapshots of yourself from another time. Remember an old issue that seemed huge then, but shows its true, less troubling colors now? You were too close-up before. That's where self-distancing changes the game. Your viewpoint shifts and, suddenly, understanding kicks in.

At times, it's like that hilarious moment in cartoons where they zoom out from an ant-sized problem made giant-sized and make-believe. When you take a step back, you'll see that intense emotion dwindle, making the **solution** a bit more reachable and less scary. This trick doesn't solve things instantly, sure, but it shrinks them towards realistic, bit-by-bit manageable size.

So, **practice**. Turn it into a habit. Anytime you feel swept away by a wave of emotions, tap into the third-person approach. Physical tools can help too—like writing things down can make stepping back a bit easier. Describe yourself, your feelings, and exactly why they're hitting you... as if writing from the view of someone else about you.

Notice the shift. The tension fizzles out bit by bit. **Decisions** seem kinder, sager, and cooler-headed. Your emotional fire gets checks from reasonable waters. Perfect for turning infernos into manageable sunsets, one distancing stride at a time.

Gaining Perspective on Personal Experiences

Think about your personal situations and **challenges** for a moment. You know how it feels when you're right in the thick of things—it can be overwhelming. You can't always see the forest for the trees. That's where **self-distancing** comes into play. By stepping back a bit, you get a wider view. It's like looking at a painting from a distance. Up close, it might just be splashes of color, but from afar, you see the whole scene.

So, how does self-distancing work in real life? Well, imagine you're dealing with a tough **problem** at work or with a friend. Instead of being stuck in the whirlwind of emotions, try to look at your situation like an outsider. What would you tell a friend going through the same thing? It's funny how much easier it is to solve other people's problems, right? That's because you're not attached to their emotions. You can see the bigger picture and think clearly.

Next comes the idea of "**temporal distancing**." Sounds complicated, but it's really simple. Think about your current problem and ask yourself: Will this matter in a week? A month? A year? Probably not as much as it feels right now. By looking at your issues from a long-term perspective, you can see that most of them are just temporary bumps in the road. It gives you a chance to focus on what truly matters in the grand scheme of things.

For instance, let's say you missed an important **deadline** at work. It feels disastrous in the moment, but if you look ahead, will this slip-up really derail your career? Probably not. It's a blip. You'll learn, adapt, and move on. Temporal distancing helps turn big, scary problems into smaller, manageable tasks.

Here's a cool technique you might like—the "**Future Self**" visualization. Picture yourself five or ten years down the road. This future version of you has wisdom, experience, and has been through what you're dealing with now. Imagine talking to them. What advice do they give you? They might remind you that you've faced similar issues before and came out stronger, or they might tell you not to sweat the small stuff.

Now, let's wrap this up by connecting these ideas. By practicing self-distancing, you start seeing your **challenges** from an outsider's standpoint. Then, you apply temporal distancing to place your issues in the context of time, which makes them seem less critical. Lastly, you use the Future Self visualization to gain insights and even comfort. Combining these techniques can make a world of difference in how you handle life's ups and downs.

Plus, it's not just about dealing with negative stuff. These methods also help you appreciate the good things in life more deeply. When you step back, look at your **progress** with fresh eyes, and anticipate future successes—you start seeing life in all its complexity and beauty. Give it a go. You might just find that stepping back brings you closer to peace of mind.

Reducing Emotional Intensity

Imagine this: **emotions** coming at you like a runaway train. You're caught in the headlights, unsure if you should brace for impact or jump out of the way. We've all been there. The trick is to create enough **distance** from those emotions so they're manageable but not suppressed. It's an art, really. Kind of like learning to drive in the rain—you don't ignore the water on your windshield; you wipe it away just enough to maintain a clear view.

Creating some distance doesn't mean pretending your **feelings** don't exist or shoving them deep down. It's more about looking at them from a different angle, like when you step back from a painting to see the whole picture instead of focusing on just a single brushstroke. Given some space, emotions lose their power to overwhelm you. They don't go away, but they become part of a larger landscape that's easier to navigate.

Next, there's something called "emotional **granularity**." Sounds fancy, right? But it simply means breaking your emotions down into more specific labels. Instead of saying "I feel bad," you might pinpoint it as "I feel disappointed" or "I feel frustrated." This way, your feelings are more like tiny, manageable grains of sand instead of a whole overwhelming desert. It's about naming those emotions accurately, so you're not swept away by a tidal wave of undefined feelings.

When you're trying to name your emotions, look for details and specifics. Is what you're feeling anger, or is it annoyance? Is it sadness, or is it nostalgia? The more precise you can be, the less intense your emotions will feel. Think of emotional granularity as giving your feelings a job title—they become easier to handle when you know exactly what they are.

Now, let's try something called "Emotional **Scaling**." It's a bit like adjusting the volume on your emotions. When things get too loud, you can dial it down. Start by visualizing yourself in two different scenarios. In scenario one, you're right there in the thick of things, feeling every slap and sting of the emotion. It's like sitting front row at a concert where the sound hits you square in the chest. In scenario two, imagine you're sitting in the back row, or even outside the venue listening from afar. The music is still there, but it's softer. Distant. More bearable.

To put this into **practice**, think of a recent emotional episode. Rate the intensity of that feeling on a scale from one to ten. Now, imagine stepping back. Maybe you're a tourist in a foreign city observing a local's outburst instead of being in the center of the drama. Picture it from a less personal perspective—a bit like watching a movie. Does the intensity drop from a ten down to, say, a seven? Six? Notice how placing some metaphorical distance between you and your emotions makes them less sharp, less hurtful.

Still skeptical? Give it a shot next time you're in the grips of a strong emotional surge. Pause and visualize yourself stepping back. Evaluate your feelings from this new vantage point. It won't dismiss your emotions, but it may help you breathe a bit easier, deal a bit better.

Understanding these **techniques** is essential, whether using the full color of emotional granularity or practicing emotional scaling. You're not just throwing emotions into a box and locking them away. You're learning to view them with a bit more kindness and distance, much like watching a storm from a safe haven—knowing it's there but not letting it tear you apart.

That painting analogy again—seeing the whole canvas instead of stressing over every individual stroke. Better yet—by practicing these methods, those once unsettling emotions might just become a vivid, yet controlled, part of your fuller picture. You're the artist after all.

And trust me, with a little **practice**, you'll get the hang of managing those emotional waves without feeling like you're constantly fighting against the tide.

Enhancing Problem-Solving Abilities

Creating some psychological **distance** can do wonders for your **brainpower** and creativity. You know how when you're too close to a problem, everything seems tangled? Taking a step back helps. Think of it like looking at a painting—when you're nose-to-canvas, all you see are blobs of color. But, when you step back, the picture becomes clear. This psychological space lets you analyze better and come up with fresh ideas.

This leads us to what's called Construal Level Theory. Fancy name for a simple idea. It suggests that things far away from you (either in time or space) are thought of more abstractly. In plain words, when something's not happening right now, you think of it in broader terms. This helps with seeing the big picture and making better **decisions**. Imagine having to decide about a job a year away. You'd probably focus on overall career goals, rather than nit-picky details like your office view. This distance helps you weigh pros and cons without the stress of immediate pressures.

So how do you actually create that distance in your head? This is where the "Wise Observer" **technique** comes in handy. Picture having an older, wiser version of yourself—someone who's gone through it all and come out just fine. When faced with a problem, think, "What would this wise version of me do?" Almost like consulting an experienced friend.

Here's a quick way to do it:

• Close your eyes for a moment.

• Imagine you're telling your problem to this wiser self.

• Visualize the advice or viewpoint they might offer.

This simple act shifts your **perspective**. You're no longer inside the problem, but looking at it from a relaxed viewpoint. Feels less overwhelming, right?

When you apply this technique, you engage parts of your brain focused on multi-angle **problem-solving**. They say two heads are better than one. In this case, it's just you... but from different angles. You'll start to notice solutions that wouldn't have popped up otherwise.

I remember a time when I was knee-deep in a work project that seemed impossible. Stress was through the roof. But when I asked my inner Wise Observer for advice, the solution seemed simple. It's weird how much your own wisdom shines when you give it the mic.

This also ties back to those analytical thinking **skills** we talked about. You're not just sitting there, staring the problem down. You're actively stepping to the side and looking at it from new angles.

So what's the takeaway here? Creating psychological distance isn't about escaping your problems—it's about shifting your viewpoint. Whether you're using Construal Level Theory to break down abstract thoughts or channeling your inner Wise Observer for sage advice, you're equipping yourself with tools to tackle issues smarter, not harder.

Try it next time you're stuck. Step back, shift your focus, and consult that wiser self within. You might be surprised how often the **answer's** right there, waiting for you to see it from a new angle.

Practical Exercise: Self-Distancing

Ever find yourself stuck in a loop, **thinking** about that frustrating event over and over again? You're not alone. We all have those moments. So let's snap out of it and try a simple **exercise** that could give you a fresh perspective. We're calling this self-distancing.

First, just think about something that's been **bugging** you recently. Maybe it's an argument with a friend or a mistake at work. Doesn't matter what it is, as long as it got you all riled up. Got it in your mind? Okay, let's keep going.

Next, close your eyes. Picture that scene as if it's a **movie** playing right in front of you. Imagine you're sitting in a theater, popcorn in hand, watching the whole drama unfold. Everything's out there on the big screen - all the words, actions, and emotions.

Now, here's the fun part. Imagine you're **floating** above the scene, like a balloon drifting up high. You're looking down at everything happening below. What do you see? How do people look from up there? Seeing things from this distance might already start to shift how you feel about it.

Let's add another layer. Describe what's happening but in the third person, using your name instead of "I" or "me". For example, instead of saying "I was upset," say "Jamie was upset." So what does this scene look like when you talk about it like that? Feels a bit weird, right? But it helps create that needed **distance**.

Okay, now think about what **advice** you'd give to a friend who's in the same situation you're in. Pretty sure it wouldn't be to stew over it endlessly, right? Maybe you'd tell them to breathe, laugh it off, or seek a solution. And there, you've started to Uncle Advice mode for yourself.

Take a minute to reflect on any new insights or **perspectives** you get from looking at it this way. Did you notice something you missed before? Maybe a small but important detail or maybe the fact that, in the bigger picture, it's not as bad as you thought. Think about these new viewpoints; they might be the keys to letting go.

Finally, write down your thoughts and any action steps you've come up with from this **exercise**. You could use a journal, a note-taking app, or even voice memos if that's more your style. What's important is getting it out of your head and into a form you can revisit later.

So, let's do a quick recap. You thought about the situation and visualized it as if watching a movie. Floating above it was next, giving you a new perspective. Describing yourself in the third person probably felt odd but helped in stepping back. Offering advice to a friend made you more compassionate to yourself. Reflecting unlocked some fresh insights. And finally, writing it all down solidified your thoughts and plans.

Self-distancing isn't about detaching yourself from your feelings or ignoring them. It's about empowering yourself to see things clearer. It's like when you take a step back from a jigsaw puzzle; sometimes, you just see where those tricky pieces fit in a little easier. So give this exercise a try, and let's see what's possible when you simply give yourself a bit of distance.

In Conclusion

In this chapter, you've discovered the **importance** of creating psychological space from your emotions. This kind of "self-distancing" can really help you **manage** your feelings and gain a better perspective on your experiences. The **techniques** mentioned, like the "Third-Person Perspective" and "Future Self" visualization, give you practical ways to apply these concepts in your daily life. When you **reduce** the emotional intensity of your negative experiences and enhance your problem-solving abilities, you're more likely to handle life's challenges effectively.

You've learned what psychological distance is and why it helps manage emotions. You've seen how **overlooking** intense emotions can improve your perspective and calmness. Quick **exercises**, like viewing yourself from a third-person perspective, can kickoff self-distancing. You've also discovered why looking at your future self makes today's problems look smaller, and cool techniques to **boost** your thinking and problem-solving.

Keep these helpful lessons in mind as you go through your day. By **practicing** what we've discussed, you can better manage your emotions, think more clearly, and tackle issues with a new level of understanding and calmness. Start trying out these techniques and see how they make a difference in your life. Stay positive and keep working towards becoming the best version of yourself.

Chapter 6: Breaking the Chains of Negativity

Have you ever felt **trapped** in your own thoughts, always dwelling on the bad side of things? I sure have. In this chapter, we're gonna break free from that cycle. Imagine stepping into a sunnier **mindset**, where you stop anchoring yourself to those self-defeating behaviors that currently bog you down.

You've been noticing those patterns, right? The negative ones that keep **looping** in your mind. This chapter guides you through understanding why they happen. Sometimes it's like your own mind is your worst enemy. Overcoming these tendencies? Easier said than done. But guess what? I'll walk you through the steps to shut down that inner **critic**.

Then, we're shifting focus to building a more positive outlook. This isn't about pretending everything is perfect but rather tweaking your **perspective** to find the good stuff more often. You'll soon realize how liberating and uplifting it can be to spot the positives even in tricky situations.

Next up, we'll get into **techniques** that give your emotions a well-deserved break. Trust me, it's like a breath of fresh air. And hey, we'll wrap up with a simple **exercise** to break those negative chains holding you back. Ready to change your **narrative**? Let's make it happen.

Understanding Negative Thought Patterns

Let's dive into what's really keeping your mind in a bad place. These are called **cognitive distortions**. Think of them like foggy glasses—everything you see is kind of hazy and off because these distortions mess with your thoughts. They give you this really twisted view of the world and keep you stuck in a cycle of bad thinking. So, let's clear those glasses.

Cognitive distortions are sneaky. They slip into your mind and make you think bad stuff is worse than it actually is. Like when you're sure you've totally **bombed** a job interview because you stumbled once. This is classic negative thinking.

And you know what? They keep you from moving forward. You get so wrapped up in these bad thoughts that you're basically frozen in place, unable to see things from any other angle. It feels like pushing a boulder uphill—immovable.

You might find yourself imagining the worst possible outcome of a situation (that's what we call **'catastrophizing'**). Ever think, "If I mess up this presentation, I'll probably get fired!" But really, one small mistake won't end your career.

And how about **overgeneralization**—where you blow one bad experience out of proportion. Like if a date went bad, and you think every future date will be a disaster. You're taking a single situation and saying it's a pattern, when it's really not.

So, how do you even spot these thought patterns sneaking in? Start by paying attention to what's going on in that head of yours. Sit back and think about that last time you felt down or anxious. What were the exact thoughts racing through your mind?

Try jotting these thoughts down. Put pen to paper and see what you wrote. Words like "always" and "never" are big red flags. "I always mess up," or "I'll never find someone who loves me." Seems dramatic, right? There's no way that's always true.

Reflecting on your thoughts this way really helps bring these distortions to light. You can see where your thinking takes a wrong turn. While doing this, you might notice other patterns too, like blaming yourself when things go wrong, even when it wasn't your fault. Or maybe you jump to conclusions faster than ever. Like, your friend doesn't reply to a text immediately and you think, "Great, they must hate me."

Keep a **diary** for a week and write down instances of negative thinking. When you see it in black and white, it's easier to challenge these distortions. Ask yourself, "Is there any actual proof that my thought is true?" or "What's a more rational view of this situation?"

Just noticing these patterns is like cleaning those foggy glasses a bit. It won't wipe them clean all at once, but it's a start. Tune into your thoughts, challenge the bad ones, and slowly—little by little—you'll stop feeling so stuck. You'll learn to let more sun in through those hazy lenses.

By recognizing you have these cognitive distortions, you gain some power over them. That boulder you thought was immovable? Yeah, it starts rolling more easily once you pinpoint those thought patterns.

So, reflect. Write it out. And **reevaluate** these things. You'll be surprised at how much clarity you gain just by checking in with your own mind.

Overcoming Self-Defeating Behaviors

You're probably familiar with how **bad thoughts** can sneak their way into your mind and play tricks on you. They can really mess with your actions. You know what I mean—moments when, even before you start something, you've already told yourself you'll fail. And what happens then? You sort of make sure it happens. It's like you're setting a trap for yourself.

This kind of thinking spins a nasty loop. Imagine a thought popping up, like "I'm terrible at presentations." The next thing you know, you're standing in front of your coworkers, already believing you'll screw up. You start fumbling, your voice shakes, and bam! You just confirmed your worst fear. That thought—that you're bad at presentations—gets stronger. Next time, it attacks again, and the cycle just keeps going. That's what they call a **self-fulfilling prophecy**. The bad thought predicts the failure, and the failure cements the bad thought.

Breaking free from that loop isn't simple. But you can do it. One powerful method is the "**Behavior Experiment**." It's a way to challenge your thoughts and prove to yourself that they're not the all-knowing truth you think they are. Basically, it's like saying to that nasty voice in your head, "Let's see what really happens, shall we?"

Here's how you can do it. You start by picking a thought you want to challenge. Maybe it's, "I'm awful at meeting new people." The next step is planning an **action** that tests this belief. You might attend a social event with an open mind, aiming to chat with at least two new folks. Keep an eye on what actually happens—do you fumble, or do you have okay conversations? Maybe you're not perfect, but guess what? You weren't a disaster either.

After the event, take some time to jot down what you noticed. Did you find new **evidence** that your initial thought wasn't completely true? Perhaps people didn't run in the other direction; maybe they laughed at your jokes or showed interest in your stories. This proves that your bad thought wasn't all-powerful. You challenge it step by step, action by action.

You might even find it helpful to create a small checklist:

• Identify the self-defeating thought.

• Plan an action to test it.

• Carry out the action with an open mind.

• Note the outcome—be truthful but kind to yourself.

• Reflect on what you learned.

Going through these steps turns theories into action. It's one thing to sit there thinking you're not great at something; it's another to actually test that theory. The more you challenge those nasty thoughts, the weaker they get. And it's empowering to see **proof** that you're not destined to fail every time.

Now, be patient with yourself. Changing self-defeating behaviors is like learning any new skill—it takes time and practice. There will be slip-ups and steps backward, but that's part of the journey. What counts is pushing forward and giving yourself space to grow.

Tackle one thought at a time with the "Behavior Experiment" approach, and you'll see gradual changes. You'll start to break that loop of negativity and replace it with truths—you are **capable**, you can succeed, and you don't need to let bad thoughts hold you back. Isn't that a fantastic revelation?

Developing a Positive Mindset

Life can throw some tough situations your way, right? It's easy to get stuck on the bad stuff, but you can flip that script. One way to do this is by **reframing** those setbacks. Instead of thinking, "Why did this happen to me?" try asking, "What can I learn from this?" It's like finding a silver lining in the cloud. Think about a time when you really messed up – maybe at work or in a relationship. Yeah, it stings. But there's always a lesson hidden in there, like a treasure hunt.

Consider how athletes often review tapes of their worst performances to figure out how to improve. They're turning their "bad" moments into opportunities for **growth**. You can do that too. The next time something doesn't go your way, see it as a learning moment – a chance for you to grow and improve. Approach each failure not as an endpoint, but as a stepping stone. Reframing helps shift your **mindset** from fixed ("I'm just not good at this") to growth-oriented ("I can get better with time and effort"). It's powerful stuff – give it a shot!

Speaking of mindsets, have you heard of learned **optimism**? It's this idea that you can train yourself to be more positive. No joke. Think of it as gym time for your brain. The process involves paying attention to how you react to situations. If you've got a habit of reacting negatively, start catching yourself – then try to find something good about the situation. It's not just about being cheerful. It affects your entire mental **health**. Optimistic folks are generally less stressed and have better emotional well-being. So, start practicing those optimistic responses and see how it shifts your perspective.

Wondering how you can practically boost that optimistic mind? Ever tried writing "Three Good Things" before bed each night? Here's the deal: every night, jot down three things that went well for you. It doesn't have to be big stuff – maybe you had a great cup of coffee or laughed at a friend's joke. Small wins count, too. Over time, it's like you're training your mind to look for positives. This **habit** gradually builds a more positive outlook and can even help lower stress.

You might think, "How do a few words scribbled on a page help?" But trust me, this little exercise can shift your focus from gloom to **gratitude**. Who wouldn't want that, right? So grab a notebook, and before you crash for the night, think about those three good things. It's such a simple but effective way to end your day on a positive note.

So, where does that leave you? Reframing negative events teaches you growth. Adopting learned optimism changes how you see the world, making you less prone to stress and more to happiness. Adding "Three Good Things" into your nighttime routine primes your mind for positive thoughts, transforming how you wake up the next day. It's these small changes that build up, making for a brighter, more positive life. Ready to give it a shot? Here's to a more positive **mindset** – one baby step at a time!

Techniques for Emotional Freedom

Bad feelings can really mess up your overall **happiness** and quality of life. Think about it. When you're constantly weighed down by negative emotions, it's hard to truly enjoy anything. Whether it's worry, anger, or sadness, these emotions can cloud everything. They mess with your relationships, your work, even your health. Sometimes it feels like no matter what good things happen, your mood still crashes and burns. That's the impact of bad feelings.

So, how do you break free from that cycle? **Emotional** control. Yeah, it sounds kind of stiff, but trust me, it's game-changing. Emotional control means being able to manage and respond to your feelings in a healthy way. It's not about ignoring or burying your feelings. Instead, it's about not letting them control your life. When you can actually manage your emotions, you find that you can face challenges without freaking out so much. Plus, being in control of your feelings means you're less likely to blow things out of proportion. Emotional control helps guide you toward emotional freedom.

Alright, let's talk about a method to get you there – the **Emotional** Freedom Technique (EFT). Imagine being able to just let go of those bad feelings weighing you down. EFT is all about using, well, **tapping**. Hear me out. You tap on specific points on your body while thinking about whatever's bothering you. Crazy, right? But it works. These points are like energy spots, similar to what you'd have in acupressure. By tapping on them, you're telling your body and mind to relax and let go.

Here's a simple way to get started with EFT:

• Acknowledge the bad feeling.

• Rate the intensity of this feeling on a scale from 1 to 10.

• Develop a reminder phrase – something short like "this stress."

• Tap on your "karate chop" point (side of hand) while repeating a setup statement, like, "Even though I have this stress, I deeply accept myself."

• Then, tap through these points while repeating your reminder phrase: top of the head, eyebrow, side of the eye, under the eye, under the nose, chin, collarbone, under the arm.

Go through the tapping sequence a few times until you notice a change in how you feel.

It might seem odd at first – tapping your head and face and whatnot. But give it a go. The tapping helps to disrupt those intense bad feelings, loosening their grip on you. You might discover your **emotional** responses start to change, becoming less intense, less overwhelming.

It's not just instant relief, though, EFT is about rewiring your reactions. Over time, with consistent **practice**, these sessions teach your mind and body to respond to **triggers** in a calmer way. It's like giving yourself a buffer against those gut-punch reactions to stress and worry.

In the end, the goal is for you to find the **freedom** where bad feelings don't have a hold on you anymore. So tap away those heavy emotions, keep those feelings balanced, and watch as your overall happiness begins to improve. Balancing emotions helps you embrace a fuller life, filled with less **stress** and more joy. Go ahead – give EFT a shot and notice the lift in your emotional freedom.

Practical Exercise: Breaking Negative Chains

Ready to **break** those bad chains holding you back? Let's dive in!

First, **identify** a bad thought or belief that frequently pops up and drags you down. It might be something like "I'm not good enough" or "I always mess things up."

Next, grab a piece of paper and create two columns. In one, list everything that makes you believe this bad thought. In the other, jot down stuff that contradicts it. Maybe you think you're not good at something, but then you remember a time you actually **nailed** it. Seeing it on paper can be eye-opening.

Now, come up with a more balanced, realistic alternative to that bad thought. Look at the evidence you've written down. There's likely some middle ground. Instead of "I'm not good enough," how about "I'm **improving** every day"? Feels better, right?

Create a positive **affirmation** that challenges your initial bad thought. Make it short and sweet, something you can easily repeat.

If your bad thought was "I always mess things up," your affirmation could be "I learn from my mistakes and get better."

Start repeating your new affirmation daily, especially when that pesky negative thought pops up. Make it a habit. Say it out loud, scribble it down, or even type it in your phone's notes. The more you repeat it, the more it'll sink in.

Keep a **diary** to note when you successfully challenge the bad thought. Jot down instances when you catch yourself thinking negatively and replace it with your positive affirmation. It'll be great to look back and see your progress.

Reflect on your feelings and actions as you keep **practicing** this exercise. Notice any changes? Maybe you're feeling a bit lighter, more grounded, less stressed. I know, it may sound cheesy, but pay attention to these shifts. They matter.

Here's a quick recap of what we've covered:

• Figure out that bad thought or belief

• Write down all the proofs that support and disprove it

• Find a balanced, realistic alternative

• Create a positive affirmation

• Repeat that new affirmation every day

• Keep a diary to celebrate your wins

• Reflect on the changes in your feelings and actions

Got it all? This exercise might feel a bit odd at first, but stick with it. Over time, it'll get easier, and you might even find it turns into a habit—a good one. Negative thoughts affect all of us, but actively working to replace them can really **transform** things. So find some time, grab a pen, and give it a go. Your mind will thank you.

In Conclusion

This chapter tackled the **concept** of breaking free from negativity, giving you valuable **tools** to change your mindset and improve your life. You've learned how to spot and **challenge** negative thoughts, as well as steps you can use to develop a more positive outlook. Changing long-held patterns takes **effort**, but the benefits make it totally worth it.

You've seen different negative thought patterns and what they look like in real life. You've also picked up ways to catch your personal negative **thoughts** through self-observation. The chapter highlighted how negative thinking can lead to unhelpful behaviors and gave you practical **exercises** to alter these self-defeating habits. You've also learned steps to convert negative thoughts into positive **affirmations**.

By putting what you've learned into practice, you've got the power to break out of negative cycles and start living a happier, better-balanced life. Take this **challenge** seriously and watch positive changes unfold over time. You've got this! Remember, Rome wasn't built in a day, so be patient with yourself as you work on rewiring your brain for positivity. Keep at it, and before you know it, you'll be seeing the world through a whole new lens.

Chapter 7: The Growth Mindset

Ever wondered what separates those who continue to **grow** from those who stay stuck? When you're faced with a **challenge**, what runs through your mind? "I can't do this," or "How can I tackle this?" This chapter is all about flipping that switch in your **brain**. Trust me, it's powerful stuff.

Think about a time you felt completely stuck. We've all been there, right? You're probably thinking, "Change is scary." Well, yeah, it can be... but it can also be the **spark** that lights up so many possibilities. You'll be amazed to see how grasping a **growth mindset** changes everything. Not only will it give you the courage to face new experiences, but it'll help you see roadblocks as stepping stones.

This idea—overcoming **fear** and reframing challenges—can transform your outlook on life. The best part? Learning to be more **resilient** and adaptable doesn't need to be daunting. There are some simple, practical steps you can try right away. By the end of this chapter, you'll likely look at **setbacks** differently.

Ready to shift your perspective? This chapter is just the beginning of tapping into new realms of possibilities you never thought were possible. Let's dive in and unlock your potential!

Understanding Fixed vs. Growth Mindsets

There's a whole **world** that Carol Dweck opens up when talking about fixed and growth mindsets. Ever notice how some people seem to take **challenges** in stride, like they're just part of the ride? That's a growth mindset. On the flip side, you've got folks who see talent or intelligence as set in stone. That's a fixed mindset.

So, what's the difference? Well, in a fixed mindset, you think your **abilities** are carved in rock. You're either good at something or you're not, period. This kind of thinking doesn't leave much room for improvement. If you fail, it feels like a dead end, 'cause you think it proves a lack of talent.

But with a growth mindset, it's like a whole other ballgame. You see abilities as something that can be developed. You aren't scared of challenges – they're just steps on the way to getting better. If you slip up, it's no biggie; it's a chance to **learn**.

Your mindset isn't just some abstract concept, though. It really shapes your whole experience - your learning, achievements, and personal **growth**. With a fixed mindset, you avoid taking risks to protect your ego. When you think your abilities are capped, why bother trying new stuff? This can leave you stuck in a rut, and ironically, not ready to deal with failure – since it feels like a wall you can't climb over.

Switch gears to a growth mindset, and it's like turning the lights on. Suddenly, challenges are exciting, like puzzles waiting to be solved. You get better at things because you actually keep at them. Struggle just means you're working towards improvement. This mindset fuels your learning, since you're open to mistakes as learning opportunities. And yeah, that means you're more likely to **achieve** stuff because you don't give up as easily.

So how do you spot the signs of a fixed mindset – in yourself or others? Here are some red flags:

- Fear of Failure: If you're always playing it safe, sticking to what you know. Avoiding risks because failure? It's because you worry it'll show your "true" limits.
- Avoiding Challenges: Blowing off harder tasks 'cause, "I'm just not good at it," rather than thinking you can figure it out.
- Being Defensive: When faced with feedback, taking it personally instead of as advice to improve.
- Resentment Towards Others' Success: Feeling envious or threatened by someone else's achievements instead of feeling inspired or seeing what you can learn from them.

Flipping that, here are signs of a more growth-oriented attitude:

- Embracing Challenges: Tackling difficult tasks and seeing them as a chance to grow.
- Learning from Feedback: Using criticism as a tool to get better, not something to take to heart.
- **Persistence**: Keeping at things even when they're tough because you know effort leads to improvement.

Spotting these tendencies in yourself takes some honesty. Just notice when you shy away from tough stuff or feel rattled by someone else's victories. Think about how you react to setbacks. Shifting towards a growth mindset isn't instant, more like changing the way you look at things over time.

It's all about transforming how you handle learning and achievements. When you start believing in yourself, thinking effort matters more than just sheer talent, things can open up. It's like giving yourself the **freedom** to mess up, take risks, and actually grow.

Overcoming Fear of Change

You might shy away from change. The known feels safe, comfy, like your favorite worn-out chair. And why **fiddle** with comfort, right? You resist change because it can be scary—it promises uncertainty and potential challenges. Plus, there's always that pesky fear of failure lurking around the corner. Unlike the predictable past, change is like an open field... unknown and, at times, daunting.

Avoiding change **stagnates** growth. If you're constantly dodging new situations, you're missing out on all sorts of chances to learn and grow. You're like a plant trapped in a small pot, unable to stretch and expand. So what happens? You end up stuck in the same place, quietly yearning for a bit more freedom. The sad part? Most people prefer this. The tight pot? It's a "safe zone." Completely eliminating risks...

But hey, that doesn't have to be you.

Seeing change as an **opportunity** rather than a threat makes it much less scary. Think of change as a new story ready to be written. No one enjoys the feeling of walking with blindfolds, but what if the other side holds something amazing? Seeing it this way shifts your mindset. It's like turning on the lights in a room you dreaded entering. Suddenly, not so bad, right?

Tips? Glad you asked:

• **Shift Perspective**: Instead of dreading the 'what ifs,' imagine the positive 'what ifs'. What if it makes you stronger? What if it opens new doors?

• Small Steps: Don't focus on the entire path. Just the next step. Like strolling rather than sprinting. One step is manageable.

• Accept Fears: It's natural to be nervous. Play friends with your fear rather than running from it. Weirdly enough, it reduces its power over you.

Now, I've got this cool method - it's called "Comfort Zone Expansion." You don't need to leap into the unknown right away. You can kind of prepare yourself gradually.

Here's how it works:

Comfort Zone Expansion

Start with tiny steps outside your comfort zone—nothing too flashy. The goal is to stretch that comfy bubble little by little until the new thing becomes, well, routine.

Steps You Can Follow:

• Daily Micro-Challenges: Do tiny, slightly uncomfortable things each day. Talk to someone new, take a different route home. No biggies, trust me.

• Reflection: At the end of each day, reflect briefly on these micro-challenges. Were they that bad? How did you manage? Each little discomfort handled makes the next one a tad easier.

• Routine but New: Add small changes into your routine activities. Drink a different coffee, read a different blog. Routine gets updated subtly which leads to less resistance.

Taking It Up a Notch

Once the small stuff feels less **intimidating**, you ramp it up a bit:

• Medium Challenges: Okay, now give the wall a nudge. Try more daring steps like public speaking or volunteering; just a one-step harder. Again, only when you are ready.

• Develop Skills: As you face more significant changes, build new skills that help you handle them better - learning can ease fear remarkably.

• Pause When Needed: Encountering resistance? Pause, don't retreat. Know it's part of growing. Above all, keep pushing.

Change isn't looking to knock you over. It's actually like a fresher breeze in a room that regrows old. When you look at change as an open-ended chance—a way for **growth**—facing it becomes much less about that scary prospect and more about the what-good-will-happen thought. Expansion of comfort zones? Helps folks not see change as a cliff, but merely a next step.

Reframing Challenges as Opportunities

Alright, let's tackle how you can flip tough situations on their heads. Instead of seeing problems as just... well, problems, what if you could see them as chances to **grow**? This small shift in thinking can change everything.

Imagine facing a tough situation. Maybe work is piling up, or you've had a disagreement with a friend. Instead of letting it weigh you down, try shifting your **perspective**. Think of these moments as opportunities to learn something new, to become stronger. Just like how your muscles grow only after you challenge them with heavier weights, your mind and heart get stronger after tough times.

Now, why does this work? When you change how you look at **challenges**, they stop being just barriers. They become moments where you learn more about yourself and your ability to handle stuff. Like when you lose a job, you might discover a passion for something new. Or when you have a falling-out with someone, you learn about what you truly value in relationships. This idea of getting stronger after going through tough times is often called "post-traumatic growth." You'll start seeing that you're capable of handling way more than you thought.

In my own life, I remember dealing with a tough breakup. It felt like my world was crumbling. But somewhere along the way, I flipped my thinking. I started focusing on what I could learn from the **experience**. Maybe I'd discover how to be happy alone or figure out what I really wanted in a partner. Those grim nights shifted into ones where I was building myself into a stronger, more understanding person. It sucks but it's also liberating.

Ready to try this out yourself? Let's get into the "Challenge Reframing" exercise. It's a simple way to practice seeing **opportunities** in tough situations. Here's what you do:

• Identify the Challenge: Pinpoint a problem you're currently facing. Maybe list out a few if you can't choose.

• Ask Questions: What can you learn from this? How can this experience make you stronger? How would someone you admire handle it?

• Find the Silver Lining: Dig deep. There's always something small you can gain. Even if it's just realizing a lesson you never want to experience again, like knowing when to set boundaries.

• Take Action: Based on your new perspective, what's your next move? Maybe it's seeking advice, trying something new, or simply, taking a breather.

For example, if you're failing a class, that sucks, right? But, in this "Challenge Reframing" process, you'd start by picking this specific **problem**. Next, you'd ask, "What can I do differently?" Maybe the lesson is time management or finding better studying methods. The silver lining could be getting to know yourself under pressure... or that you need help and it's okay to ask for it. Finally, act on this.

Find a tutor, create a study group, or even speak to your teacher about extra help.

Changing how you see problems isn't a magic fix. It's training your **brain** to focus on the positive side. And it does take some time. But with practice, you can begin seeing these so-called 'problems' as spots to grow.

By reframing challenges as opportunities, you put yourself on a path to handle life's curveballs with more grace and **wisdom**. Don't expect perfection. Small steps are still steps forward, leading you to a place where you're not just surviving... but thriving. Isn't that worth the effort?

Developing Resilience and Adaptability

Wanna know a secret? Building **mental toughness** and staying **resilient** starts with really simple steps. Mental toughness is all about keeping you steady when life throws punches. It's like the backbone of a growth mindset, solid yet flexible.

Think of it as having a sturdy, inner shield. When setbacks come along, instead of crumbling, you stay strong. Focus on these key parts:

• **Self-Belief**: Your inner cheerleader. You know you've got what it takes to push through tough times.

• Motivation: The drive that pushes you forward — yeah, even when you don't feel like it.

• Emotional Regulation: Keeping cool. No meltdowns, just calm, steady waves.

• Focus: Blocking out those nasty distractions. Staying on the path.

• Resilience: Yep, bouncing back, no matter what happens.

When you practice these, your growth mindset thrives. This means you see challenges as chances to grow, not brick walls.

Life never sits still. Everything's always shifting — careers, relationships, personal goals. You gotta be **adaptable** to succeed and stay happy in such a spinning world. Imagine water flowing smoothly around rocks. That's you, adapting to life's twists and turns.

Being adaptable isn't just nice—it's vital. Think about it. When plans change — which they always do — adaptability helps you stay on course. Instead of panicking or feeling defeated, you tweak your approach. You stay fluid. It lets you see challenges as problems to solve instead of hurdles to trip over.

Now, let's jump into building that resilience. There's a cool trick to make your emotions and mind more flexible. Here's one to hang on your mental fridge – it's called "**Bounce-Back Visualization**."

Picture this: Think of a time you faced something tough but got through it. Replay that in your mind. Close your eyes. Feel that strength, that grit. This trick rewires your brain to be better prepared for future challenges. It's like mental muscle memory. You train yourself to see difficulties and immediately think, "I got this."

Want another nugget? Stay **curious**. You know how kids keep asking "why" until they're satisfied? As adults, we lose that sometimes. If you stay curious about your failures or stumblings, like "What happened there?" and "How can I twist this into a win?" you'll figure out ways to turn mishaps into opportunities.

Let's jam on control too. Focus on what you CAN do, rather than what you can't. Shifts your mental energy to something constructive. Balancing all this makes you resistant to stress.

All of this – mental toughness, staying flexible, building resilience – pours into your ability to adapt. So when things don't go as planned, you spring forward, ready for whatever's next.

The magic happens when you mix them all up. Keep **practicing**. Keep **pushing**. Your mind will learn to dance in the storm, finding joy, growth, and freedom without getting bogged down.

Practical Exercise: Adopting a Growth Mindset

Alright, here we go — adopting a **growth mindset** is an adventure, kinda like stepping into new shoes that might feel a bit awkward at first, but soon you'll be running comfortably. Let's break it down into manageable steps, making it simple and actionable.

First, spot that fixed belief. Look at your life and find an area where you're set in your ways. We all have them. Maybe it's your career, relationships, or even a hobby. Pick just one, the one that bugs you the most. How do you normally think about this part of your life?

Next, write down your thoughts. Grab a pen and paper — or type it up if that's more your speed. Jot down what you believe and feel about this area. Be honest, raw even. This isn't for anyone else's eyes but yours. It might look something like, "I'll never get better at this," or "It's just not for me." Whatever it is, lay it bare. It's like dumping everything from an overcrowded drawer onto the floor so you can see it all.

Now, **challenge** those beliefs. Play detective. Look at each of those fixed ideas and start questioning them. Ask yourself if there's proof you can grow and improve. Has there ever been a time when you, or anyone else, actually did get better in this area? Search for those cracks in the wall where light seeps through. Maybe you recall a time when you improved, even slightly. Or perhaps you came across someone who did. Challenge those rigid thoughts.

After that, create **growth-focused** statements. Flip those old beliefs on their heads. Write down new ones – statements that focus on growth. For example, instead of "I'm terrible at this," write, "I can get better with practice," or "This is a skill I can learn." Do this for each fixed belief. It might feel weird at first, kind of like trying to speak a new language, but that's okay. Change takes practice.

Then, set a small **goal**. Pick one related to the area you're focusing on. But keep it small; something totally doable that nudges you a bit outside your comfort zone. If it's a project you feel stuck on, commit to spending just 10 minutes each day working on it. Or, if it's a social thing, maybe try starting a conversation with someone new.

While working towards that goal, focus on **learning**. Zoom in on what you're learning, not just ticking off the outcome. Pay attention to your progress, however small it may be. Every tiny step counts. This shift, from focusing on the end result to the learning journey, can be huge.

Finally, reflect on your **progress**. Maybe do this after a week. Write down how you felt doing the exercise, what you learned, and what surprised you. Did you discover something new about yourself? Did you see even a slight improvement? It's all about celebration, however small the victory may seem.

By following these steps, you've taken a concrete, actionable path towards adopting a growth mindset. It's those baby steps that make all the difference. Keep at it, and before you know it, you'll think about that old fixed belief and realize it's like those old shoes you outgrew — pretty soon, it'll be hard to imagine you ever felt that way.

In Conclusion

In this chapter, you've delved into the **importance** of having a growth mindset and how it can **transform** your approach to learning and facing challenges. Understanding the differences between fixed and growth mindsets helps pave the way for personal **development** and resilience. By viewing challenges as opportunities and overcoming the fear of change, you can achieve significant **progress** in various aspects of your life.

You've seen that fixed and growth mindsets are two different ways people approach learning and challenges. Your mindset affects how well you do in school, sports, and other activities. Signs that you or others might have a fixed mindset include fear of making mistakes. Being scared of change can stop you from growing, but seeing change as a chance can help. **Techniques** like the "Comfort Zone Expansion" can ease you into accepting change.

By applying what you've learned in this chapter, you can start making small daily **changes** that add up to significant improvements over time. Always remember that with a growth mindset, the sky's the limit! Try to see every obstacle as a new way to get stronger and smarter. Keep **practicing** these ideas, and you'll be amazed at what you can **accomplish**!

Chapter 8: Silencing the Inner Critic

Have you ever had a pesky little voice in your head telling you you're not good enough? Yeah, I've been there too. It's that **annoying** inner critic. In this chapter, I'm aiming to quiet that voice for you, once and for all. Yep, I want you to face and **challenge** all those self-limiting thoughts and start seeing yourself through kinder, gentler eyes.

You know when that **negative** self-talk sneaks in, making you second-guess everything you do? Well, that stops here. You'll learn to spot those bad patterns and **reframe** them in a way that actually helps you thrive. Think of it like cleaning out the clutter in your mind.

You don't need to be a superhero to show yourself some **compassion**. This chapter is chock-full of tips to help you feel nicer and more patient with yourself. Trust me, it's like getting a hug when you really need it.

And oh—don't miss the **practical** exercise at the end. It's a game-changer and will guide you in **transforming** that inner dialogue for good. Together, we'll unleash a more **confident**, less critical you.

Identifying Negative Self-Talk Patterns

You know that **annoying voice** inside your head that just won't give you a break, right? That's your inner critic. It's like having your own personal heckler following you around, smashing your **confidence** and self-worth at every turn. Where does it come from, you ask? Well, this unwelcome guest generally checks into your life during childhood.

Think back to early life experiences. Maybe a teacher scolded you once. Perhaps you tried hard to win a school race but came last, and someone teased you for it. Little things to one person can be big mountains to another. These moments leave a mark and soon shape how you talk to yourself. Over time, you start internalizing those criticisms until they morph into your regular thinking. Your once carefree mind turns into a fertile field for this self-doubt.

So, how do you catch these thoughts? Let's talk about some common types. For instance, there's "all-or-nothing thinking." This little bad boy makes you see everything in black and white. One tiny slip-up at work? Well, you're a failure, end of story. Or how about "taking things personally"? Someone passes you without saying hello, and your mind starts spiraling – "What did I do wrong?" or "They must not like me."

There's more. How about "**catastrophizing**"? One small hiccup, and suddenly, your brain's convinced the sky is falling. Miss a deadline? You're already visualizing getting fired and living under a bridge. Or let's not forget "labeling." You make a simple mistake and boom, suddenly you're slapping a permanent label on yourself: "I'm such an idiot." See the trend? These thoughts aren't doing you any favors.

Now, it's time to spot these pesky voices in your daily life. Here's what you could do. Start keeping a little diary, not one where you scribble all day, but just jotting down spots where these bad **thoughts** pop up. Say you made a mistake at work and your brain went haywire. Write down exactly what you thought and why it might not actually be true.

Pay attention to how you feel. Start noticing **patterns**. Often feel anxious when meeting new people? Maybe you're struggling with thoughts like "They won't like me" or "I'll mess up and say something dumb." Or do you dread feedback at work fearing "I'm never good enough"? Spot those feelings and trace them back to the thoughts fueling them.

Meanwhile, be patient with yourself. Seriously, you aren't changing overnight. This self-analysis is like training a puppy. It requires consistency, kindness, and a bit of humor might help. Someday you'll catch a thought, roll your eyes, and think, "Oh, there's my inner heckler at it again." That's **progress**.

Don't shy away from asking for support. Sometimes talking to friends or relatives you trust can provide an outside perspective. They're not stuck in your head, so they can often see what you can't.

In simpler words, you're looking for habits here, trying to shift the **script** you use to talk to yourself daily. It's about catching the usual suspects of negative self-talk lurking in corners and throwing them under the light. With time and practice, you'll start recognizing these negative patterns more quickly.

Next, you gotta work on getting rid of them, but that's another chapter for another time. For now, just know you're stepping on the right path. You're ready to quiet that inner critic and turn its volume way down. Neat, right?

Challenging Self-Limiting Beliefs

You know those **thoughts** that say you're not good enough or you don't deserve success? They can really hold you back from growing and achieving what you want. These pesky self-limiting beliefs make you second-guess everything. Instead of focusing on what you can **accomplish**, you get stuck worrying about what might go wrong. So, how do you kick these thoughts out of your head? Well, challenging them is a good place to start.

One way to do this is by using cognitive restructuring techniques. That might sound all technical and complicated, but it's pretty simple. It just means changing the way you **think** about things. Start by identifying your self-limiting beliefs. Write them down and look at them. It's like shining a spotlight on the villain in a mystery movie.

Once you've found your limiting beliefs, question them. Ask yourself stuff like "Is this really true?" or "Do I have evidence to back this up?" Most of the time, you'll find that these beliefs are just unhelpful stories you've been telling yourself. They're not based on facts. Now that you've questioned these beliefs, the next step is to **reframe** them.

Reframing is kind of like taking a picture that's crooked and straightening it so it looks better. For example, if you keep thinking, "I'm terrible at public speaking," you can reframe that thought to be something like, "I can get better at public speaking with practice." See the difference? One thought is limiting and makes you feel like there's no point in trying. The other one opens the door to improvement.

Okay, so we've tackled questioning and reframing. How about the "Evidence Gathering" method? Pretty neat concept. Think of this as a way to play detective with your own mind. You're on a mission to find **evidence** that disproves your limiting beliefs. Let's break this down.

Say you think you're not smart enough to get a promotion at work. Gather evidence against that belief. Maybe you got good grades in school or you have successfully completed challenging projects in your current job. Write all this evidence down. When you see the facts laid out like that, it's a powerful way to start believing in yourself more.

It's also helpful to get outside opinions, like from a friend or mentor. They often see things you miss. They can provide examples of times when you've been successful or shown great ability. They might say, "Remember when you led that big project on short notice and did a great job?" That's evidence, too.

Here's a little story for you—imagine you've been limiting your **career** options because you believe you aren't good at networking. Through evidence gathering, you realize you've actually made several key connections in the past. Perhaps at a conference or even through social activities. These instances act as proof that you aren't as bad at networking as you thought.

After gathering all this evidence, review it whenever you feel those limiting beliefs creeping back in. Over time, this new way of thinking can become **habit**.

So there you have it. From questioning and reframing your limiting beliefs to the "Evidence Gathering" method, these steps can help you break free from those pesky thoughts holding you back. It won't happen overnight, but with a bit of practice and perseverance, you'll start to see change. And that's pretty **empowering**.

Developing Self-Compassion

You might wonder how being kind to yourself differs from having high **self-esteem**. It's a fair question. High self-esteem is about feeling great based on your accomplishments and seeking external validation. It's like saying, "Look at what I've done, I'm **awesome** because of it." But it can be shaky because when you don't succeed or get that praise, your self-worth takes a hit. On the flip side, **self-compassion** is about treating yourself kindly no matter how you're doing. You mess up? No biggie. You're kind to yourself regardless. This kind approach leads to better **mental health** because you don't tie your worth to success or failure. You're cool with yourself even when things aren't going so well.

Self-compassion has three parts. Three simple yet powerful parts:

• Being nice to yourself. This means talking to yourself the same way you'd talk to a good friend. Imagine your friend messes up; you'd likely say something comforting or supportive, right? Do the same for yourself. Negative self-talk can be a downer, so switch it up and give yourself a break.

• Realizing you're not alone in your struggles. Everyone messes up. Seriously, everyone. It's easy to think you're the only one, especially in today's world where everyone puts their best moments online. But you're not alone. When something goes wrong, know that other people are going through similar stuff. It's like this invisible bond that connects all of us. This part of self-compassion helps you see your struggles in the larger human context. You're part of a tribe, buddy.

• Being **mindful**. This is about being aware of your feelings without getting all wrapped up in them. It's like observing your thoughts and emotions without judgment or overreaction. When you feel bad, notice it but don't start thinking the world is ending. Just be present in the moment and acknowledge how you're feeling without making it worse by overthinking.

So, how do you respond kindly when things get tough? Here's where the "**Self-Compassion Break**" comes in. This exercise is pretty simple and really effective. You can use it whenever you're stressed or feeling down.

First, pause and take a few deep breaths. Relax. Then, say to yourself, "This is a moment of suffering." Recognize that you're going through a hard time. Allow yourself to feel it. Next, remind yourself, "Suffering is a part of life." This helps you remember that you're not alone. Finally, place your hand over your heart or give yourself a gentle hug and say something kind like, "May I be kind to myself," or "May I find peace."

This whole exercise takes just a minute or two, but it's like a reset button for your **emotional state**. You're not brushing away your feelings; you're acknowledging them with kindness. This can be hugely comforting and can really shift how you're feeling.

And there you have it. Being kind to yourself isn't the same as just trying to boost your ego. It's this sustained, compassionate mindset that helps you through the ups and downs. And, with the Self-Compassion Break, you've got a handy tool to tap into whenever life's being a bit rough. So go easy on yourself. You're doing just fine.

Reframing Negative Thoughts

Switching up the way you **think** can really change your life. It's like taking off dark shades and putting on clear ones. The world doesn't change, but the way you see it certainly does. You might've been caught in this loop of bad thoughts, thinking everything's your fault or nothing's going your way. Sound familiar? Well, guess what? You can actually change that.

Being mentally **flexible** means not sticking to one viewpoint. Imagine you're in a rigid bubble and, sometimes, stuff squeezes in and makes that bubble super tight and uncomfortable. But if you're flexible, your bubble can stretch and bend. It can accommodate new ideas and different perspectives. You get to look at things from all kinds of angles.

It's kinda like how you might look at **art**. You could be looking at one piece and see sadness, while someone else sees beauty. Both views can coexist, right? Changing how you look at situations in life, especially the tough ones, can bring the same kind of clarity.

Your problem might not be as massive as you thought. Maybe that mistake you made isn't the end of the world.

Here's where the "Thought **Reframing**" technique comes in handy. Think of it like this: you find yourself thinking, "I messed up that project, I'm such a failure." Stop. You catch the thought in action, sort of like catching a foul ball. Now, instead of letting it hit you, you throw it back—reframe it. Maybe try saying, "I didn't do great on that project, but I learned something valuable, and I can do better next time."

It's like having a mental **toolkit**. You reach in, pull out a tool, and start tinkering with those thoughts. You don't just accept the negative as gospel truth. Instead, you question it. Ask yourself: "Is this thought helping me? Is it even accurate?" Often, thoughts like "I'm always screwing up" aren't really based on facts. They're exaggerated and not useful.

Think of these reframed thoughts like patches on a bicycle tire. You fix the leaks and you're able to get **moving** again, smoothly and confidently. This practice, over time, makes positive thinking almost automatic. It turns into a habit. And before you know it, your mindset shifts, just like that.

Sometimes you might think, "I can't do this," and all you need to do is tweak it a bit to something more balanced, like, "This is hard, but I can try it and see how it goes." This isn't about pretending everything is amazing. It's about balancing the negative with realistic, helpful thoughts.

Look, nobody is saying it's easy. It takes some **effort**. But once you start, you'll notice how much lighter you feel. More hopeful, less weighed down by negativity. It's as though you've been carrying a heavy backpack and someone just took a bunch of bricks out.

The next time you catch yourself spiraling into bad thoughts, stop and give reframing a shot. Your **mental health** will thank you. This little shift can have a massive impact on how you feel every day.

Sort of like changing the radio station from static to your favorite song. Give it a try—your clearer, happier self is waiting.

Practical Exercise: Transforming Self-Talk

Pick out a **negative thought** you keep saying to yourself. You know the one. That mean thought that always cuts you down. Let's say it's "I'm just not good enough." Everyone's got one (or a few), so grab one of your greatest hits.

Jot down the **feelings** you get from this thought. How does it make you feel? Really crappy, right? Maybe it brings on sadness, frustration, or even fear. Whatever it is, write it down. Be honest with yourself.

Look at the **evidence** for and against this bad belief. Break it down. What facts do you have that really back this up? Maybe you messed up on a project once or twice. But what about the other times you kicked butt? Often, there's way more against these beliefs than for them.

Come up with a more **balanced** statement instead. This part is super important. Take that rough thought and flip it. Not into something unrealistically positive, but something true. Maybe something like, "I have strengths and weaknesses, but I try my best."

Say the new **statement** out loud whenever that bad thought pops up. This may feel a little weird at first—like you're talking to yourself. But this is a game-changer. When "I'm not good enough" enters your brain, counter it with, "I have strengths and weaknesses, but I try my best."

Think about how saying the new statement changes your **feelings** and **actions**. Does the new thought make you feel a bit lighter? Less weighed down? It can help you act less out of fear and more out of confidence. Seriously, take note of this.

Keep doing this with other negative thoughts you notice. You've tackled one but why stop there? There's bound to be more. Identify those other critics in your head and put them through the same process. The more you practice, the better you get at it.

This **exercise** doesn't fix everything overnight, but it guides you toward kinder self-talk with small, manageable steps. And that's pretty much the goal—to be kinder to yourself, one thought at a time.

In Conclusion

This chapter has given you **valuable insights** and **tools** to silence that nagging inner voice that often puts you down. You've learned about recognizing and challenging your negative thought patterns, why **self-compassion** is so crucial, and practical steps to change the way you talk to yourself. These lessons are vital for building a healthier **mindset** and a more positive self-perception. Let's wrap things up with the key takeaways.

You've discovered the importance of spotting when your inner critic takes over and why it usually stems from early life experiences. You've also learned about common negative thinking styles like all-or-nothing thinking and taking things too personally. Recognizing these patterns daily can help you start to see the influence of your inner critic.

You've explored ways to question and change self-limiting beliefs that hold you back from achieving more. You've also picked up practical methods to help transform negative self-talk into kinder, more realistic statements.

Applying these lessons can help you build a kinder relationship with yourself. Why not make a **commitment** to not let your inner critic hold you back? Start practicing these **techniques** daily, and watch as your inner dialogue shifts positively. Take the **courageous** step forward; you truly deserve to silence your inner critic and grow into the best version of yourself!

Chapter 9: From Perfectionism to Excellentism

Ever **wondered** why chasing perfection feels more like a trap than a path to improvement? You might have. You get caught up in every tiny flaw, and suddenly, you're stuck. But guess what? There's a way out.

In this chapter, you'll embark on a **journey**. You'll discover a new mindset where mistakes are just stepping stones, not the end of the world. Forget **punishing** yourself for not being perfect; that's old news. Instead, you'll learn how to set realistic and healthy **standards** that keep you moving forward – not spinning in circles.

Imagine **learning** without that nasty self-judgment whispering in your ear. You'll leave those harsh inner critics at the door and get cozy with a **growth-oriented** mindset. And you know what's cool? There's a practical **exercise** waiting for you – making Excellentism not just an idea but a reality you can practice right away.

So, as you kick back and dive into this chapter, get ready to trade in perfectionism for something a whole lot more awesome. **Intrigued**? You should be – your next steps might just surprise you in the best way possible.

Understanding the Pitfalls of Perfectionism

Ever wondered what's the deal with **perfectionism**? How's it different from just aiming high? When you're setting lofty goals, you're pushing yourself to grow, like training for a marathon to get stronger. But perfectionism? It's like expecting to win that marathon on your first-ever run. Totally unrealistic, right?

Instead of motivating you, perfectionism traps you in a cycle of never feeling good enough. The **mental toll** is huge. Picture that nagging voice in your head, always unsatisfied, telling you that you could've done better no matter how hard you tried. That really messes with your mental health, leading to stress, anxiety, and even depression. You might find it hard to enjoy anything, always fretting about flaws and mistakes. And let's not forget about sleep—or lack thereof. You're tossing and turning all night, replaying every little error in your mind. Wake up tired and cranky, and the whole miserable cycle starts over.

Your **body** doesn't get off easy either. Stress hormones go through the roof, jacking up your heart rate and blood pressure. It's like you're on a treadmill you can't stop. Constantly chasing an impossible standard burns you out—fast. You get headaches, feel exhausted all the time, and might even weaken your immune system, making you more likely to get sick.

Ever notice how you end up **procrastinating** when you're trying to be perfect? Weird, isn't it? You'd think a perfectionist would be super productive. But nope. The fear of not getting something absolutely right can paralyze you. You'll spend so much time planning and refining that you never actually get started. Or, if you do start, you keep going back to redo and refine, rather than moving forward.

Napoleon famously said, "Perfection is the enemy of the good." It's like this with **decisions**, too. You can't make them quickly because you're scared of making the wrong one. So you stall or analyze every possible outcome—and get stuck. This puts you off from trying new things or taking risks. You don't achieve much because, well, you're still planning how to achieve much... forever.

Also, think about those times you managed to finish something. Was it satisfying? Or were you immediately worried about what could be better? That's the thief of **joy** right there. Accomplishments should feel good. They're steps on your personal journey, but perfectionism turns these milestones into burdens.

Over time, this pattern follows you everywhere. **Work** becomes a series of stressful, overwhelming projects. Home life gets tense, too, because you're imposing the same impossible standards there. Perfectionism doesn't stay contained in one part of your life. It spreads pretty fast.

It's a tough **habit** to break. Admitting things are "good enough" rather than "perfect" takes practice. It's about letting yourself slip up sometimes and move on. Accepting you can't control everything focuses your energy on what matters. You're here to grow, not to be flawless.

So there you have it. Striving for excellence keeps you motivated. Perfectionism? Not so much. It exhausts you, holds you back, and robs your joy—far from the freedom you truly deserve.

Adopting a Growth-Oriented Mindset

Imagine shifting from perfectionism to something called excellentism. It sounds funky, but stick with me. The **idea** here is about targeting excellence while dodging the stressful, nit-pickiness of being a die-hard perfectionist.

Perfectionism has its nest in chasing flawless results. It's like setting yourself up for disappointment—over and over, you'd cling to unrealistic standards. But why not focus on excellentism? It's about **striving** for excellence without getting tangled up in the nitty-gritty of perfection. You'd aim for high standards but allow for mistakes, which can often be more beneficial in the long run.

Now, if you're cool with that, let's talk about a **growth-oriented** mindset. This is when you're more about learning and improving rather than sticking to some unchanging standard. It's like being a learner rather than a knower. The difference is subtle but powerful. With a growth mindset, you know you won't be perfect, but you will get better. Bit by bit.

How does switching from being a perfectionist to having a growth-oriented perspective help you achieve excellence? For starters, you won't be paralyzed by the fear of making mistakes. Mistakes become **learning** opportunities. Yeah, a bit cliché, but also true. You're moving forward, iterating, improving. That's the way you aim for excellence without the downsides of perfectionism. You release the need to be spotless and instead focus on being the best version of yourself at any given time.

Switching gears a bit, here's the method—Progress over Perfection. It's your ticket out of the stress of trying to meet unrealistic standards. Progress over Perfection is about valuing the little steps, giving yourself credit for moving forward, no matter how small the steps might be.

So how do you start aiming for **progress** instead of total flawlessness? Simple:

• Celebrate Small Wins: Give yourself a pat on the back for small accomplishments. It makes a big difference in keeping up your motivation.

• Set Smaller Goals: Breaking tasks into bite-size pieces makes them more manageable, and each completed piece gives you a win.

• Reflect and Learn: When things don't go as planned, instead of freaking out, take a breather. Think about what went wrong and how you can do better next time.

And suddenly, you're obsessed with improving and growing, which is way cooler and less stressful than being a perfectionist. You worry less about being error-free and more about how you're better today than yesterday. It's a shift in focus from unachievable perfection to achievable **growth**.

So here's the kicker—as you embrace excellentism and a growth mindset, you'll find that you actually **achieve** more. Why? Because you're more flexible, more adaptive. Less likely to burn out. More likely to get up when you stumble and keep moving forward. You're building an excellent you, one small win at a time.

I get it—change isn't easy, especially if you've clung to perfectionism for years. But adopting a growth mindset and focusing on progress can lead to less stress, more achievements, and most importantly, a happier you.

It's a **journey** worth taking, huh?

Setting Realistic and Healthy Standards

You know what trips a lot of people up? The difference between having high standards and setting unrealistic expectations. It's like this: high standards **push** you to be your best, while unrealistic expectations set you up to feel, well... defeated. High standards are **motivating**, but when your expectations are way out there, they end up doing more harm than good.

Imagine you've got a kid in school. You want her to get good grades. That's a high standard. Now, demanding she scores an A+ in every test, joins all the clubs, and never makes a mistake, that's just not fair. It's setting her up to feel she's never enough. Same goes for yourself. Set high but achievable **goals**, something that pushes you to grow but doesn't stretch you too thin like a rubber band ready to snap.

Why set goals focused on the process? Good question. When you're only chasing the end result, you miss out on the **growth** that happens along the way.

Take running a marathon for example. If you're only obsessed with finishing, you might push yourself to the point of injury. But when you focus on the training, the small victories, and the improvements, it becomes more about enjoying the ride rather than just crossing the finish line. You learn to appreciate the process, enjoy the little wins, and even if things don't go as planned, you've gained skills and had some fun on the journey.

Speaking of goals, there's this handy method called "SMART Goal Setting." Ever heard of it? If not, I'll fill you in. SMART stands for Specific, Measurable, Achievable, Relevant, and Time-bound. It's like a reliable friend guiding you through your goal setting process.

Here's how it works:

• **Specific**: Instead of saying "I wanna be healthier," go for something like "I wanna jog three times a week." More clear.

• Measurable: Make it something you can count. Like, "I'll write 500 words a day." That way, you know when you've met your goal.

• Achievable: Sounds great to say you wanna move mountains. But aim for goals that are realistic, given your time and resources. "I'll learn to cook one new dish every week," is better than aiming to become a gourmet chef in a month.

• Relevant: Make sure your goal ties into who you are and what you truly want. If learning a new hobby doesn't interest you, pick something that does.

• Time-bound: Set a deadline. Saying "someday" often means "never." Aim to "complete a 5k run in three months," and it gives you a timeline to work with.

When all these elements come together, your goals don't seem like massive hurdles. Instead, they become actionable **steps** you can see yourself conquering. And let's be honest, ticking off those small victories feels enormously more satisfying.

So, next time you're setting a goal, or feeling the weight of that pressure to be perfect, try dialing it back a bit. Aim for **excellence**, not unattainable perfection. And enjoy the process of getting there.

It's a smoother ride when you're not constantly worried about the end result. Plus, you get to celebrate every little **win** along the way. And that, in itself, is pretty motivating, right?

Learning from Mistakes Without Self-Judgment

Wanna know a secret about **perfectionism**? It can totally stop you from learning. Always wanting to be perfect means you're basically scared to mess up. And when you're scared to mess up, you don't try new things. You don't take risks. You spend all your time worrying about doing everything right that you never actually get better at anything. It'll box you in a corner, stalling progress and making you more stressed than doing your math homework on a Sunday night. Yup, being too hard on yourself can be a hell of a buzzkill.

But **mistakes**—oh, the good ol' mistakes—are actually pure gold when it comes to learning and growing. Think about it. Each mistake shows you what didn't work. It's like seeing a sign that says, "Don't go this way!" And the more you notice those signs, the more you know what paths to steer clear of. Hitting a wall can teach you more than breezing through can. Pretty crazy, right? Mistakes and setbacks aren't the end of the world; they're clues in your treasure hunt. The inconveniences that pop up can guide you to where you need to go, as long as you're looking at them with the right sort of lens.

So how do you pick out the nuggets of wisdom in all that mess without tearing yourself to pieces mentally? That's where the "Mistake Analysis" trick comes into play. It turns blunders into **learning** opportunities instead of self-flagellation tools. Here's how it works:

First, pause. Take a breath. Seriously. Step back from the situation to see it from a distance. Any strong emotion—disappointment, embarrassment, frustration—needs to be caught first. Then, acknowledge you made a mistake, but skip blaming yourself. "Yeah, this happened. What now?" Next, evaluate the mistake objectively. What went wrong? What was the trigger? Get the facts. After that, identify the lesson. What can you take from this so you don't repeat it? It can be something tiny, like adjusting your note-taking method, or big, like realizing you need more prep time. Finally, plan forward. Think of what you can do next time instead. Make a plan, but remember, it doesn't need to be foolproof.

With the Mistake Analysis trick, there's no harsh self-talk or saying things like, "I can't believe I did that." **Compassion** is key here. Because the goal isn't about one-off perfection, it's about continuous improvement—closer to "excellentism" than perfectionism. Like aiming for a balanced middle where you do well enough without exhausting yourself.

It can be like trying to eat healthier. You won't always pick the salad over pizza, but when you occasionally do, that's progress. Practice combining kindness with analysis—finding a mix that works best for you. Listen to your own needs.

Shift away from perfectionism and start viewing mistakes as stepping stones, rather than dead ends. Making room for these "mistake opportunities" fosters **growth**, naturally moving you toward better outcomes without the stress perfectionism brings. Effectively turning self-judgment into self-encouragement. Got it? Cool. Now, you've got a roadmap to turn your slip-ups into **success**.

Practical Exercise: Excellentism in Action

Pick a task or project where you usually **aim** for perfection. You know that thing you always want to get just right? Maybe it's a work presentation, organizing your home, or even a hobby. Choose one and stick with it.

Now, set a realistic, time-bound **goal** for this task, focusing on progress rather than perfection. Aim for something achievable in a set amount of time. Instead of trying to make your presentation flawless, aim to have it done in three days. Be honest about what's doable.

Break the task into smaller, manageable **steps**. Think of this as turning a mountain into a series of hills. For that presentation, you could break it into researching, creating slides, and practicing. Smaller steps mean less overwhelm and better focus.

For each step, decide what "good enough" looks like. This one's a bit tricky but important. What's the minimum needed to get the job **finished**? For researching, maybe three solid sources are enough; for slides, they should be clear—not perfect. Deciding what "good enough" looks like can save you tons of time and stress.

Set a time **limit** for each step to avoid over-editing or too much revision. The temptation to keep tweaking things can be strong. Setting a time limit means you move forward. So, give yourself an hour for research, two for slide-making, and so on. Stick to it. You can always tweak more later if absolutely necessary.

After finishing the task, reflect on what you learned and how you **improved**. Maybe you notice that working with clear steps makes you feel less stressed. Or you realize that "good enough" really was good enough—it got the job done, perhaps even better than striving for perfection.

Celebrate your **progress** and finishing the task, no matter if it's perfect or not. It's important to celebrate—even if it wasn't perfect! You made progress, you got it done—a win's a win. Maybe treat yourself to something small or just take a moment to savor the fact.

In doing this exercise, see how each step feeds into the other. You're setting yourself up for less stress and more **progress**. The shift from always aiming for perfection to focusing on excellentism can be a game-changer—less weight on your shoulders and more joy in your achievements. Got a task in mind already? Start small, focus on these steps, and watch how things get better without needing to be perfect.

In Conclusion

Chapter 9: From Perfectionism to Excellentism offers **valuable insights** and practical advice on letting go of perfectionistic pressures and embracing a healthier approach to achieving excellent results. It emphasizes the importance of adopting a **growth mindset**, setting realistic goals, and learning from mistakes without beating yourself up.

In this chapter, you've discovered the difference between healthy striving and harmful perfectionism. You've learned about the personal and professional **costs** of chasing unrealistic standards and how perfectionism can actually make you **procrastinate** more. The chapter introduces the positive, growth-oriented mindset of excellentism and guides you in setting achievable, process-focused goals instead of unattainable ones.

You'll find **practical strategies** for shifting from being perfect to being excellent by prioritizing progress and learning from experiences. Remember, pursuing excellence with realistic expectations is far more **meaningful** and attainable than striving for flawless achievement. Go ahead and apply these principles to different aspects of your life, and you'll find yourself **growing**, learning, and achieving more in a balanced and fulfilling way.

So, why not give it a shot? Embrace excellentism and watch how it transforms your approach to challenges and goals. You might be surprised at how much more you can accomplish when you're not tied down by the chains of perfectionism. It's time to **excel**, not perfect!

Chapter 10: The Practice of Nonattachment

Have you ever felt trapped by your own **expectations**? I know I have. That feeling when things don't go to plan can be so frustrating. In this chapter, we're tuning into something that might just shake things up for you—**nonattachment**.

Imagine feeling at **peace**, regardless of what happens. Sounds too good to be true, right? Well, hang in there. This chapter isn't about getting rid of your desires but learning how to let go of clinging to the results. Think of it like loosening the grip on a rope—suddenly, the pressure starts to ease.

I've spent years figuring out how to release the hold of expectations. You'd be amazed at the **calm** that comes when you finally do. You'll pick up ways to stay emotionally **flexible** when life throws curveballs and find peace even when things change. It's not about being indifferent; it's about being free from the chains of rigid outcomes.

Plus, there's this cool **exercise** that'll show you how to actually practice nonattachment. Curious yet? Good. Come along and discover how letting go can feel strangely **empowering** in this ever-changing world.

You're about to embark on a journey that'll teach you how to roll with the punches and find your **zen** in the chaos. It's all about learning to go with the flow without losing your cool. You'll see how loosening your grip on those iron-clad expectations can actually open up a whole new world of possibilities.

Think of it like surfing. Instead of fighting against the waves, you'll learn to ride them. It's not about giving up on your goals, but rather about being **adaptable** enough to navigate the twists and turns life throws your way.

Ready to dive in? You've got this! Let's explore how embracing nonattachment can be your secret weapon in staying cool, calm, and collected, no matter what life dishes out.

Understanding the Concept of Nonattachment

You're diving into the idea of **nonattachment**. You might think it's just another term for detachment, but they're quite different. Detachment often means cutting off feelings or distancing yourself emotionally. Picture someone cold, indifferent. They don't really engage with their emotions or even people around them. It's like putting up walls.

Nonattachment, on the other hand, means **accepting** and feeling your emotions but not letting them control your life. It's like acknowledging a cloud that passes by but not clinging to it. You feel it, you see it, and then you let it go. You don't hold onto the outcome of situations, whether good or bad. This is totally different from detachment, where you don't feel anything at all.

Imagine you're in a situation where you're tied to an outcome. Maybe you're really hoping to get a **promotion** at work. You put all your energy into it, and when it doesn't happen, you're crushed. It seriously sucks. This attachment to outcomes sets you up for disappointment. It also keeps you from growing. You become so focused on one result that you miss out on other opportunities. You might even hunker down, afraid to step out and try again. It's like having tunnel vision, and it's pretty limiting.

On the flip side, practicing nonattachment can really help you build **resilience**. When you stop clinging to a specific outcome, you're free to explore other paths. You accept whatever comes your way. Sure, you may feel sad or disappointed for a little while, but those feelings don't control you. You're like bamboo that bends with the wind but doesn't break. It's a kind of flexible strength.

When you're nonattached, you're more emotionally **stable**, too. Your mood isn't dictated by external events. Lost that promotion? Okay, what's next? You learn to move forward without that weight dragging you down. It's like putting on emotional armor but without cutting yourself off from the world. You still engage fully, just without letting it weigh you down.

I remember a time when I was applying for universities. I'd put all my hopes into one specific school, thinking it was absolutely the only place for me. Spoiler alert: I didn't get in. It was devastating initially. But once I stopped obsessing over that one setback and opened my eyes to other possibilities, things got way better. I ended up going somewhere else, making fantastic friends and finding opportunities I never even dreamed of at that 'perfect' school.

Having nonattachment helps with your **relationships**, too. You're no longer putting unrealistic expectations on others. You're not trying to control how things should go. You let the relationship flow naturally. If a friend cancels plans, you're like, "Okay, no biggie," rather than sulking all day. This kind of attitude makes you easier to be around and, believe me, people notice.

To wrap it all up, nonattachment doesn't mean you stop caring. It means you care without becoming **fixated**. You're free to move through life more smoothly, less rocked by every little bump. Think about it like hiking. You enjoy the path, not just the view from the peak. You're **adaptable**, more resilient, and honestly, much happier. Time to lace up those emotional hiking boots and hit the trail.

Letting Go of Outcomes and Expectations

Focusing on the **process** instead of the results can be great for your mental health. Picture this: when you're just enjoying what you're doing and not obsessing over what might happen, you can actually live in the moment. You know that saying, "it's the journey, not the destination"? Well, there's truth in that. By paying more attention to what you're doing right now, whether it's a project at work, a hobby, or even a workout, you're more likely to enjoy yourself. You can also handle **stress** better because you're not constantly worrying about whether or not you'll succeed.

When you have strict **expectations** about how something should turn out, it can make life a lot harder. They can set you up for a world of stress. Think about it. You spend all this time imagining how things should be and then when they don't go your way, it's like a mental smack in the face. You feel disappointed and let down. Realizing that not everything will go your way or be perfect can save you a lot of headaches.

Now, how do you let go of these preset ideas? Here's an "**Expectation Release**" trick that might help. Basically, whenever you catch yourself stressing over how something is supposed to turn out, stop for a second. Ask yourself one simple question: What will happen if things don't go exactly as planned? Most of the time, the answer is, "nothing horrible," or "I'll be okay." Once you recognize that, it becomes easier to shift focus back to the process instead of the outcome. Just like that—poof—you start to stress less.

Another part of the trick is to practice a bit of **mindfulness**. Find a quiet moment and think about recent situations where you had a lot of stress because things didn't go as you expected. Remind yourself how, in the end, everything worked out okay, even if it wasn't perfect. You can even go a step further and actually write these examples down. It's sort of like giving yourself proof that, hey, it's not the end of the world if things don't go exactly as planned.

You can also talk to yourself in a supportive way. Instead of saying, "It has to turn out this way," try saying, "I hope it goes well, but I'll be fine if it doesn't." It might sound simple, but changing your inner dialog can make a big difference. Through **self-talk**, you can become your own coach, cheering yourself on and minimizing the pressure you feel.

Another thing that can help is sharing your worries with someone you trust. Sometimes just saying out loud what you're stressed about can make it seem less intimidating. You're putting it out there and it loses its power over you. Plus, talking it out can give you new perspectives on how to deal with stress and expectations.

In general, it's back to focusing on the **process**. When you're enjoying the journey and not focused on how it's supposed to end, each moment becomes more fulfilling. This can lead to a happier, less stressful life. So next time you find yourself caught up with outcomes and **expectations**, just take a step back and breathe. Enjoy what you're doing for the sake of doing it. That's where real freedom lies.

Developing Emotional Flexibility

Imagine you're in the middle of a really **stressful** day. Your boss just piled up more work, you got stuck in traffic, and to top it off, you had an argument with a friend. Yeah, pretty chaotic. But what if being emotionally **flexible** could help you handle all this better?

See, emotional flexibility is about staying cool and **adapting** to whatever life throws your way. It's kinda like yoga for your feelings. It helps big time when you're up against stress. When you're emotionally flexible, you don't freeze or freak out. Instead, you bob and weave, making it easier to find ways to cope. It's like having a rubber band heart—it stretches under pressure but snaps back when things go back to normal.

But it doesn't just help with stress. Your **relationships** get better, too. Think about it: When you're able to roll with your emotions, you're less likely to snap at people. Your patience grows. Your empathy increases. This kind of flexibility lets you hold space for others without letting their stress rub off on you. You get to be that balanced friend who listens without judgment and supports without being drained.

Now, let's talk about something called emotional **agility**. It sounds fancy but really, it's just another way of describing how you adapt to changes. Life's full of twists and turns, right? Bad days, good days, and meh days, too. Emotional agility is about staying open to all those experiences without letting any single one define you. You acknowledge your feelings—especially the tough ones—without letting them control you.

Think of it like this: Emotional agility is a dance. You see the music change and you switch your moves. Instead of resisting the flow, you dance along. This ability avoids those emotional brick walls we sometimes hit when things don't go our way. It makes the tough days less brutal and the good days even sweeter.

So, how do you get better at this? One exercise I really like is "Emotional **Surfing**." Yeah, it's about riding the waves of your emotions without wiping out. Picture yourself on a surfboard. Feelings are like waves. Some are small ripples, some are massive tsunamis. Emotional surfing teaches you to stay balanced. Here's how it works:

• Notice the Wave: Pay attention to what you're feeling. Is anger bubbling up? Or maybe sadness? Just name it.

• Stay on the Board: Don't jump off. Let yourself feel whatever it is without running away or suppressing it.

• Maintain Balance: Focus on your breath. Slow, deep breaths. Picture yourself balancing on that board.

• Ride it Out: Feel the emotion as it peaks and ebbs away. Trust that every wave settles eventually.

By practicing Emotional Surfing, you give yourself the freedom to feel **emotions** without being overwhelmed. It's like giving your emotional self the same freedom you give your physical body to roam. You're going with the flow, knowing that waves come and go, and none of them last forever.

Getting good at this takes practice but man, is it worth it. It brings a lot of peace and helps you stay centered when everything around you is chaotic. Plus, it makes your interactions with others a whole lot smoother.

In the end, being emotionally flexible and agile isn't just about handling stress or connecting better with people. It's about enjoying life without getting bogged down by it. You'll find it easier to appreciate the little things and not waste energy on the stuff that tries to drag you down.

So, go ahead, ride those **waves**. Your emotional surfboard is waiting.

Finding Peace in Impermanence

You know, the idea that everything **changes** can feel a bit scary at first. But once you accept that things don't last, you start seeing the world differently. Instead of stressing about losing what you have or what's coming next, you become more **present**. It's kind of freeing—learning to appreciate moments and experiences as they come, knowing they're temporary.

Because things aren't forever, it makes the good moments shinier and lets you handle the tough ones better. Think about it; when you're sure that hard times aren't permanent, it gives you a weird kind of **strength**. It's almost like saying, "This too shall pass." Really, it makes each day feel like a little gift, doesn't it?

When we talk about dealing with life's uncertainties, there's this concept called "radical **acceptance**." It's not just any kind of acceptance—it's diving deep and really getting okay with what's happening, even the stuff you really don't like. Sure, it's easy to accept the good stuff, who wouldn't? But it's the not-so-great things that are the real test. Radical acceptance is about saying, "Alright, this is what's here right now, and that's okay," without trying to change it or wish it away.

This doesn't mean you roll over and let life do whatever it wants. Not at all. Instead, it's about facing life head-on, acknowledging that you can't control everything. It's kind of like accepting the weather—you'd no sooner shout at the rain to stop or the sun to shine. You accept it and figure out how to live with it. This stops you from getting tangled up in **frustration** and helps you move through life with a bit more ease.

Now, how do you get yourself to that level of acceptance? Well, there's this cool technique called "**Impermanence** Reflection." Sounds fancy, but it's really simple. Basically, you take some time each day to think about the impermanent nature of life. Yep, that's it. Could be during a walk, when you're in line at the coffee shop, or just lying in bed at night. You ponder how everything, both good and bad, is always shifting and changing.

This reflection makes it easier to let go of stress about the future and regrets about the past. You're training your mind to be flexible, to flow with life's ups and downs instead of fighting them. It's like you're building mental muscles for acceptance and **adaptability**.

Life's a whole lot easier when you aren't holding on so tightly to things. When you remind yourself that everything is part of this ever-changing river, you can navigate life's rapids better. It's quite the relief, right?

So really, finding peace in impermanence isn't about giving up or resigning yourself to whatever happens. It's more about flowing with life, embracing its changes, and finding a sense of calm in that flow. You start to see that each **moment**, whether joyful or challenging, has its place. And that makes it a whole lot easier to enjoy life, free from the clutches of overthinking and regrets.

Practical Exercise: Practicing Nonattachment

Alright, let's dive into this. Nonattachment isn't about not caring; it's about finding **peace** no matter where things lead. So how do you practice it?

First, think of a **goal** or desired outcome you're super attached to. It could be getting that promotion at work, buying your dream house, or finding your soulmate. Whatever it is, jot it down.

Now, let's talk expectations...

Write down all the expectations and **assumptions** you've got tied up with this goal. Perhaps you think getting that promotion will make you happier, more respected, or secure. Maybe you're assuming that buying the house will finally give you that sense of adulthood you crave. Really let it all out here; be honest with yourself.

Look at each expectation. Imagine some different ways things could play out. Maybe getting that promotion means more stress and less time with your family. Maybe another home shows up in a few months that's even better. The point here is that your path could twist in all sorts of ways. Think of plan Bs and Cs instead of laser-focusing on Plan A.

Find parts of the whole **process** that you can actually enjoy, regardless of the outcome. Like, even if you don't get the promotion, are there elements of your current job you can appreciate? Or, while house-hunting, can you enjoy exploring different neighborhoods? This gets you to extract joy from steps instead of just looking at the finish line.

Now, create a **mantra** or affirmation. Something that grounds you in the present and eases up on that crazy focus on the end result. Try, "I enjoy the journey and embrace where I am right now." Doesn't have to be that exact phrase, but something that works for you.

Make it a **habit** to repeat this mantra every day. Especially when the anxiety strikes and you're stressing over how things will turn out, take a breather and repeat your phrase. Consistency matters here.

Take a moment to **reflect**. See how shifting your focus impacts your stress levels and how much you're actually enjoying the ride. You might find you're less wound up about the outcome and more at peace with where you are.

Think about it, shifting your viewpoint seems small, but it can really ease your mind. Suddenly, the journey itself has value. Instead of life being a series of finish lines, each step along the way holds something worthwhile.

So run through these steps as often as you can. Pick a goal, jot down those expectations and assumptions, imagine other outcomes, find enjoyable parts in the process, create that mantra, repeat it daily, and reflect on the whole change. It's like training for a marathon, start slow, and pretty soon nonattachment becomes second nature.

There, you've got it. Practicing nonattachment doesn't uproot your core but transforms how you relate to your **pursuits**. Pretty soon, you'll feel lighter, less trapped by outcomes and more liberated to live.

In Conclusion

In this chapter, you've delved into the **practice** of nonattachment, getting a guide on how to manage your **emotions** and expectations more effectively. This technique is a game-changer for your well-being, helping you lead a happier life despite life's roller coaster ride. By shifting your focus from specific outcomes to the journey itself, you can dial down the **stress** and soak up the present moment.

You've learned the ins and outs of nonattachment, including:

• The key difference between nonattachment and detachment in emotional and psychological contexts

• How being hung up on outcomes can lead to suffering and put the brakes on personal growth

• The way nonattachment boosts your **resilience** and gives your emotional well-being a lift

• The major psychological perks of zeroing in on the process rather than the result

• How rigid expectations can pile on unnecessary stress and set you up for disappointment

By putting these ideas into action, you can grab the reins of your **emotions** and live a more fulfilling life. Why not start practicing nonattachment today? You'll be amazed at the peace that comes from letting go of your need for specific outcomes. Take these

lessons and use them to navigate life's twists and turns with grace, turning each day into a chance to learn and **grow**.

So, what are you waiting for? Dive in and start applying these **insights** to your daily life. You've got this!

Chapter 11: Rewriting Negative Self-Scripts

Ever wonder why those old, critical voices keep **echoing** in your head? Well, I did too. I realized that those harmful self-scripts were like bad roommates—they refused to leave and messed up my mental space. But here's something you should think about: What if you could **kick** them out and rewrite those scripts?

In this chapter, you'll find the keys that'll open doors to a whole new way of seeing yourself. I promise, it'll be worth it. Imagine **recognizing** those nasty patterns that drag you down and flipping the script on them. Ever thought about how your stories shape your life? You'll learn some cool techniques to take **control** and turn those bad stories into empowering ones. And guess what's next? Reinforcing those positive beliefs so they stick.

Oh, and I've included a practical **exercise** to fix your self-script. It might sound daunting, but it's actually kinda fun. Believe me, it's easier than you think. Before you know it, you'll build a **narrative** that lifts you up instead of bringing you down. Let this chapter spark your **curiosity** and get you ready to see changes. Trust me, you're on the edge of something **amazing**.

You're about to dive into a world where you can reshape your inner dialogue. It's like giving your mind a makeover, and you're the stylist. Get ready to toss out those worn-out thoughts and replace them with shiny new ones that'll have you feeling like a million bucks. So, buckle up and get ready for a wild ride through your own psyche.

Recognizing Harmful Narrative Patterns

Ever **think** about how you talk to yourself in your head? Those little stories you tell yourself about who you are and what you're capable of? They're called self-scripts, and they shape everything—from your **behavior** to your self-image. It's like having a narrator in your brain, but not always a friendly one.

Self-scripts are these internalized stories. Sometimes they're helpful, nudging you to be your best. But other times, they can be downright nasty. If your script is "I'm always messing things up," that's going to affect how you tackle a new **project**. Spoiler: Not very confidently. You start hesitating, doubting yourself—and guess what? You end up messing up, creating a self-fulfilling prophecy.

Common negative self-scripts can leave you feeling like you're trapped in the same old movie. There's the "victim" script, where you think everything bad happens to you and there's nothing you can do. Then there's the "imposter" script. Sound familiar if you think you don't deserve your successes and keep waiting for someone to declare you a fraud? High-achievers often feel this way—like they've just managed to trick everyone into thinking they're competent.

Spotting your own negative self-scripts is the next step. It's a bit like tuning into a radio station on an old-fashioned dial. You have to get past the static before the voice becomes clear. Start by paying attention to your thoughts, especially when you're feeling low. What exactly are you saying to yourself?

Let's say you've just had a rough day at work. You find yourself thinking, "I'll never get things right," or "I'm so useless." Bingo! You're hearing a harmful narrative pattern. It's easy to ignore these thoughts because they feel so automatic. But take a minute to write them down. When you see them on paper, they often look exaggerated or downright untrue.

Picking up patterns means noticing when these same scripts pop up time and again. Do you feel like an imposter every time you start a new project? Maybe you always play the victim when **relationships** don't work out. Recognizing these repeated stories helps you figure out where they're coming from. Are they echoes of things you've heard from family or bosses? Past failures and criticisms turned into a cassette that keeps looping?

So, how do you own those scripts and start making **changes**? Reflect. Ask questions like, "Is this thought really true?" and "What evidence do I have to support it?" Sometimes, you'll find the script is based on absolutely nothing solid. For instance, if you think you're always messing up, list moments where you didn't. You'll realize you have wins under your belt.

Remember, it's not just about spotting these patterns but **challenging** them. Rewrite those scripts one step at a time. Switching "I'll never get it right" to "I'm learning and improving" can be transformative. Speaking to yourself more kindly, as you would to a friend, actually changes the script and, over time, the outcome.

These scripts love staying hidden, twisting reality and pushing self-doubt. But by tuning in, spotting the patterns, and slowly rewriting them—you'll kick those harmful narratives to the curb. Sound tough? It can be, but it's one of the most powerful ways to free up some mental space and maybe, just maybe, start feeling like the **star** of a much better movie.

Techniques for Cognitive Restructuring

So, you're about to dive into cognitive restructuring and how it helps change those pesky thought patterns stuck in your head. Sounds **complicated**, right? But it's actually pretty straightforward. Think of cognitive restructuring as a way to fix your thinking. It's like spring cleaning for your **brain**. You go through all the cluttered mess of bad thoughts, reorganize them, and toss out what doesn't serve you anymore.

Cognitive restructuring is a big part of cognitive-behavioral **therapy** (CBT). Basically, it involves identifying those bad thoughts that are messing up your mood and behavior, challenging them, and changing them into something more positive and helpful. So instead of letting a bad thought spiral into a whole dark cloud of negativity, you catch it, question it, and turn it around into something a lot more encouraging.

One key model in CBT that helps with cognitive restructuring is the ABC model. Here's an easy way to remember it:

A. Activating Event - Something happens. Like, your friend doesn't answer your text right away.

B. Belief - What you think about the event. Maybe you think, "Oh, they must be mad at me."

C. Consequence - How you feel or what you do as a result of that belief. You end up feeling anxious or even sad.

If you think about it, the same event can cause different reactions based on your belief. If you change the "B" – the belief – you change the "C" – the consequence. Like, instead of thinking your friend is mad, you might think they're just busy. Different belief, different outcome. You won't feel bad anymore because the new belief is way more reasonable.

So, how do you get good at this? Well, one useful **tool** for this process is the "Thought Record" method. It's like having a diary but for noting down specific events and analyzing your thoughts.

Here's a simple way to start a Thought Record:

• Situation: Write down the actual event. Like, "Friend didn't answer my text."

• Mood: Note how the situation made you feel. Was it anger, sadness, worry? And rate its intensity (like on a 0-10 scale).

• Automatic Thoughts: List whatever immediate thoughts popped into your head. Stuff like, "She hates me," or "I must've done something wrong."

• Evidence Supporting Thought: Whatever reasons you think support that bad thought. But be honest – is there any real evidence?

• Evidence Against Thought: Challenge with facts that don't support the bad thought. Like, "She's been great with texting back before," or "It's only been ten minutes."

• Alternative Thought: Come up with a new, more balanced thought. Something like, "She might just be busy with something."

• Outcome: Now that you have a new thought, check how you feel. Did your mood improve? Do you perceive the event differently?

This method runs you through a step-by-step to figure out why you're feeling a certain way and gives you a chance to consciously correct it. Regularly using Thought Records will help you catch and fix those bad thoughts before they rule your life. Practice makes perfect, you know?

It's like finding that **mirror** into your beliefs and flipping those detrimental scripts. Over time, this can become second nature, and you'll find your mental state much lighter and more freeing.

All in all, mastering cognitive restructuring requires **practice** and patience. Remember, it might feel a bit odd at the start, but trust me

- with time, it's worth it. Just keep at it and take it one thought at a time. Results will follow.

So, there you go. That's the lowdown on cognitive restructuring, the ABC model, and the Thought Record method. Keep exploring, keep questioning, and you'll see positive **changes** happening in no time.

Creating Empowering Personal Stories

Hey there! Have you ever thought about the **stories** you tell yourself? You know, those ones where you focus on what went wrong instead of what went right? It's easy to get caught up in all the bad stuff, isn't it? But what if you could **reframe** those stories to showcase your strengths and resilience? Let's talk about how you can start doing that.

The stories we tell about our lives shape how we see ourselves. This is what psychologists call "**narrative identity**." It's basically how we understand who we are through the stories we tell about ourselves. When you focus on the bad stuff, you end up with lousy self-esteem and low motivation. Flip that around, and it's a game changer!

Now, think about the **obstacles** you've faced. Tough jobs, broken relationships, health issues—every twist and turn. What if instead of seeing these as failures or setbacks, you started seeing them as your training grounds? Let's make those training grounds the highlights of your story. For example, instead of saying, "I failed at my job," how about, "I learned valuable lessons in a challenging work environment"?

It makes a huge difference if you focus on how you came out on the other side. It's not about ignoring the struggles; it's about highlighting how you've **grown** because of them.

Let's talk about the "**Hero's Journey**" for a sec. Imagine your life as a movie. You're the main character—your own hero. In these kinds of stories, heroes always face challenges. They go through hardships, meet mentors, and come out stronger. So why not cast yourself as the hero in your own story?

Here's how you can do it. Start with where you were. Paint that picture. Maybe you were in a tough spot, didn't see much of a way out. But did you give up? No, you fought back. You picked up the pieces. That's stage one—the call to adventure, if we're thinking Hero's Journey.

When you hit the struggles, you didn't just sit there, right? You actively looked for ways to **improve**, sometimes hesitatingly, sometimes boldly, but you took steps forward—maybe learning new skills, seeking advice, making tough decisions. This can be your 'road of trials'—lots of smaller challenges preparing you for the big win.

You've got to love those little wins. No matter how small you think they are. Each one stacks up to bigger things. Celebrate those. Share those in your story—with yourself and with others. Folks love a good comeback story, and it's as motivating for you, the narrator, as it is inspiring for the listener.

Now fast forward to today. You've gathered wisdom, strength, and **resilience**. This is the stage where you stand tall. Tell that! Imagine talking to a friend; you wouldn't leave out your hard-earned victories, right? So, don't leave them out when you're talking to yourself.

Before we wrap up, make a habit of picturing your life story the way these elements blend together. The startup, the trials, the transformation zones, and finally, your standing ground. You get the point?

In short, leave room to tell a better version of your life's story. One that showcases you as the resilient hero. One where every downturn is just another scene in a compelling movie. Speak highly of your struggles—they're badges of honor. And the best part? You wrote your script.

Reinforcing Positive Self-Beliefs

Let's **chat** about why you should even think about reinforcing positive thoughts. Your **brain's** a bit like a field. Keep walking the same path, and you make a track. That's how your brain works with thoughts. If you're always going down negative thought paths, that's what gets reinforced. But when you start treading down positive ones, you carve out new, healthier tracks. Important, right?

Think of this process like choosing to plant flowers instead of weeds. When negative thoughts pop up, they're like weeds that take over if you don't pluck them. Positive thoughts? They're your flowers. By focusing on the good stuff, you nurture these flowers, creating a beautiful, thriving **garden** in your head. And who doesn't want that?

Self-affirmation. You've got to hear about this. It's saying good things about yourself to yourself. Sounds simple, but trust me, it's **powerful**. By repeating positive statements like "I am capable," or "I deserve love and respect," you actually start to believe them. These affirmations can do wonders for your **confidence** level and your performance.

Ever noticed how athletes psych themselves up before a game with positive talk? "I'm the best. I've got this." It reprograms their mind. You can use self-affirmation in the same way. When you keep saying positive things about yourself, over time, your brain accepts them as truth. This boosts your confidence, making you perform better in whatever you're doing, be it work, relationships, or personal goals.

Now, let's discuss a nifty little tool called the "Positive Evidence Log". Like a diary, but instead of just jotting down your thoughts, you record instances that prove your positive self-beliefs.

Maybe it's making a great point at a meeting. Jot it down. Got a compliment on your cooking? Write it up. Helped a friend through a rough patch? Add it to the list. By gathering all this positive **evidence**, you actively fight those pesky bad thoughts that say you're not good enough. Over time, you have this growing log of awesome things you've done, making it easier to counteract those bouts of doubt we all sometimes face.

Imagine, at the end of the week, flipping through your positive evidence log. You see all these little (or big) wins. It's an amazing confidence booster. Instead of your brain defaulting to negative self-scripts that got ingrained over time, you have a bunch of real, positive facts staring you in the face. Makes it kinda hard to say, "I can't do this," when you've got all this proof that, yep, you totally can.

Look at these **methods** as tools you can use every day. They're not just random acts; they become a gentle routine in your life. Over time, reinforcing positive self-beliefs isn't just an activity—it becomes who you are. Like planting those flowers, eventually, you end up with such a lovely garden in your mind that the weeds don't stand a chance. You stroll through life, and that self-confidence shines.

And, might I add, feeling good about yourself starts reflecting in how others see you too. Which means **opportunities** come your way, and you start enjoying your relationships and work more. It's a win-win.

Practical Exercise: Self-Script Revision

Ever catch yourself saying the same, tired story in your head? Like, "I'll never be good enough," or something in that vein? We all have these pesky **narratives** that just refuse to leave. It's like they're stuck in your mind, playing on a loop. The trick here is to grab one of those nagging tales and take a good look at it. Maybe it's about never feeling smart enough, or always thinking you're going to mess things up. Got it? Great. Let's go a bit deeper.

Get out a piece of paper or your journal and write it down. All the nitty-gritty details. Every negative whispered lie you've been telling yourself. When did it start? What do you **believe** about yourself because of it? How does it make you feel? Hurt, sad, angry? List those feelings too. It's almost like getting it out in the open so you can deal with it. Seeing it all on paper makes it real but also manageable.

Right, now take another look but with a skeptical eye. Does that story really hold water? Can you find any **evidence** that contradicts it? Maybe someone told you that you did a fantastic job on a project or you passed that tough test with flying colors. Gather all those instances where life said you're not your negative story. Sometimes, we overlook the good stuff, so dig a little.

Time to rewrite. Write down a new tale that aligns with who you want to be, instead of who you're afraid you are. If your old story was "I'm terrible at public speaking," maybe your new story is "I'm learning to be more **confident** in sharing my ideas." This new story should vibe with your goals and beliefs. Make it positive and hopeful. Not perfect, just better and truer to the real you.

How can you support your shiny new story? Whether it's taking a class, practicing a skill, or even just talking kinder to yourself. Write down a few **actions** you can take to live this new narrative. If part of your story involves learning better communication, maybe your action is to join a local speaking group or reach out to friends more often.

Now it's time for repetition. Every day, spend a few minutes saying your new story back to yourself. Look in the mirror if it helps. **Visualize** moments where you can see yourself thriving in this new story. It's a bit like giving your brain a friendly reminder—it takes some time and practice, but you'll get there.

Get another journal or just flip to a new section of your current one, and jot down your little wins. Each time you live out your new tale, write it down. These entries become your personal 'proof' that the new story isn't just wishful thinking—it's happening. And you're making it **happen**.

So there you go, a practical exercise to flip the **script** on negative self-talk. Like I always say, it all starts with catching these little buggers and writing them down. The power of change lies in turning the page, quite literally. Give it a go and see what unfolds.

In Conclusion

This chapter has offered valuable **insights** on how to rewrite negative self-scripts to change your **mindset** and improve your life. By recognizing harmful narrative patterns, applying cognitive restructuring techniques, creating empowering personal stories, reinforcing positive self-beliefs, and revising self-scripts with practical exercises, you can **transform** the way you see yourself and your potential.

You've learned about what self-scripts are and how they **impact** your thoughts and actions. You've explored different types of negative self-scripts, like feeling like an imposter or always being the victim. You've discovered ways to identify your personal negative self-scripts by reflecting on your thoughts and noticing patterns.

The chapter has also equipped you with **strategies** to change negative thinking using methods like the ABC model and Thought Record. You've learned steps to create new, positive stories about yourself and build **confidence** every day.

By incorporating these **techniques**, you're not just challenging negative thoughts; you're paving the way for a more empowering and positive life. If you apply these methods consistently, you'll soon see a remarkable **transformation** in your self-belief and mindset.

Remember, changing your self-scripts is a journey. It takes time and practice, but the results are worth it. Keep pushing forward, stay positive, and watch as your new, empowering narratives shape a brighter future for you!

Chapter 12: The Journey of Forgiveness

Ever felt like you're lugging around a hefty backpack crammed with **grudges** and pains? This chapter is gonna be the beacon you need to ditch that burden. You might be wondering if **forgiveness** can truly offer a fresh start. As someone who's been down this road, I can tell you - it absolutely can.

Picture yourself **letting go** of past hurts and moving forward with a lighter heart. This chapter aims to guide you through understanding what forgiveness is really all about. It's more than just uttering, "I forgive you." It's about a shift in how you **feel** and think. And believe me, you won't be going it alone - I'll be sharing some personal stories to help you connect.

We'll dive into the four Ds - the simple steps you can follow. Bit by bit, you'll uncover **self-forgiveness** too, finding that sweet inner peace. By the time you're done, moving forward won't just be a pipe dream, but a totally doable goal. And yeah, there's even a hands-on exercise thrown in - a **forgiveness letter** you can write. It's not just something you'll skim over, but something you'll actively take part in.

Intrigued yet? You're in for a life-changing read, one that might just be the key to a lighter, **brighter** future. Get ready to embark on your own journey of forgiveness and discover the freedom that comes with letting go.

Understanding the Nature of Forgiveness

Forgiveness, in the field of psychology, isn't just about saying "it's okay" or making up with someone. It's way deeper than that. It means letting go of **anger**, resentment, and the wish for revenge. It doesn't mean you forget or excuse the wrongdoing, but you choose to release the negative emotions tied to it. Imagine it like clearing out an emotional closet; you're not stuffing it down or forgetting about it, but making space for better things.

When it comes to forgiveness, you'll go through a journey of feelings and steps. It all starts with recognizing there's something to forgive. You feel the hurt and maybe even hate. Ask yourself why holding onto this hurt isn't helping. It feels heavy. Then, you have to decide to forgive. This isn't saying what happened was okay, but rather saying, "I'm done letting this control me." You might feel a bit conflicted here because letting go can feel tough. Next, start working on **empathy**. Try to understand why the person hurt you. Not so you can excuse it, but so you can sort of see them as human, with their flaws and all. You'll probably feel lighter here, and maybe just a bit more at ease.

As you forgive, remind yourself this process is for you, not them. This helps foster your **emotional** well-being. You see, hanging onto past wrongs builds stress, anxiety, and even sadness. Letting go of this baggage, you start to feel a lift—a clearer mind without the clutter. The person you're forgiving benefits too—knowing they are forgiven surfaces relief, a clean slate. But believe me, the mental boost you get feels way better.

Shifting attitudes can ripple through your whole **mindset**. For me, forgiving someone was like shedding old skin. I felt new, kinda like I'd given myself permission to live lighter. And yeah, it's work. It's not some magic moment where all's forgiven and forgotten. It's little steps and a heap lot of introspection.

Think of this as cleaning up whenever someone says something hurtful or lets you down. Note how stressed out and tired it makes you. Holding **grudges** lets that person take space in your head without any rent. Forgiving them boots them out and reclaims that room for peace and joy. Finally, it's motivational in relationships. It not only fixes old bonds but builds a way stronger foundation.

So, forgiving is really about understanding and moving past hurt. It's releasing toxic **emotions** for your own betterment. Does it sound overly simple? Sure, but easy? Nope. Yet, it brings mental peace worth all that effort. It's an action for your **healing** and well-being. Just keep this mantra, "Forgiving isn't forgetting. Forgiving is **freedom**."

The Four Ds of Forgiveness Process

Let's chat about the Four Ds. They really help you **navigate** forgiveness in a way that's simple yet effective. These Ds stand for Decide, Deepen, Do, and Deepen Again. Don't sweat it, though – it's easier than you might think.

First, you've got to **Decide**. This is when you make up your mind that it's time to forgive. You finally say, "That's it, I'm done holding onto this hurt. I'm choosing to let it go." It's that kind of firm, line-in-the-sand decision we're talking about. Without this, the rest of the process crumbles. So, you need to nail this stage. Think of it as the foundation of your whole forgiveness journey.

Then you **Deepen**. This stage is about digging a bit deeper (don't worry, it's not another deep dive). You take a moment to understand the why. Why did this sting so much? What's behind it? Maybe there's old baggage there, stuff that's been weighing you down. You look at the core of the pain and really acknowledge its impact on you. This step makes it real, and trust me, that's crucial.

Next, you move to **Do**. This stage puts those insights into action. It's about expressing your forgiveness – both to yourself and, if it feels right, to the other person. A super powerful way to do this? The "Forgiveness Letter" technique. Basically, you write a letter to the person who hurt you, but you don't have to send it. You pour out all those bottled-up feelings and then declare your forgiveness. Seeing your emotions on paper is almost therapeutic. It's a physical act that reflects an internal decision.

Finally, you've got to **Deepen** Again. Yeah, you're revisiting all that emotional excavation. But it's about renewal this time. Almost like cleaning out the last bit of junk. You look at how you've grown, how much lighter you feel, and acknowledge what you've learned through this forgiveness process. You kind of layer this new understanding back into your daily life, solidifying your decision. It's reinforcement, ensuring that forgiveness isn't just a one-time thing.

So, these four steps form a cycle – you might find yourself going through them more than once. And that's totally normal. Forgiveness isn't necessarily a one-and-done deal.

To put the "Forgiveness Letter" technique into perspective, imagine this: you sit down with a pen and paper. Start writing to the person who hurt you. Be brutally honest about your feelings. Write everything out. Then, declare your forgiveness. Say "I forgive you, and I release this anger" – or whatever feels right for you. Remember, you're not sending this letter, so go ahead, pour your heart out. When you're done, you might even want to do something symbolic, like ripping the letter up or burning it. Something physical to match that emotional release.

This Four Ds framework makes sure you cover all bases – from decision to action, and back to deeper reflection. It's a loop designed to help you fully let go. So next time that past hurt pops up, you've got a clear path to work through it. Just stick to the Four Ds and watch your emotional **burdens** get lighter.

Self-Forgiveness and Inner Peace

Forgiving yourself is a tricky business. It's not the same as making excuses for your actions. When you make excuses, you're brushing off responsibility, saying, "I did that, but it wasn't really my fault." But when you **forgive** yourself, you're accepting what happened—you did what you did. Then, you choose to release the **guilt** that's weighing you down. It's a massive step toward emotional healing. You can't move forward if you're stuck in the past, holding onto every mistake like a heavy bag from a shopping spree gone wrong.

The difference lies in the **accountability**. Making excuses means running away. Self-forgiveness means facing it head-on. You say, "Yeah, I messed up, but I'm choosing to learn and let go." It's a game-changer—a pathway to **peace**. When you're constantly blaming yourself, you build a wall between you and your happiness. Tear it down, brick by brick. Give yourself permission to be human.

This brings us to self-compassion. It's all about being kind to yourself. If you treat a friend who's made a mistake with understanding and kindness, why not do the same for yourself? Self-compassion is like being your own best buddy who's got your back. It's reminding yourself that everyone messes up. It's okay to be imperfect. You replace harsh self-criticism with a gentle, nurturing voice. Think of self-compassion as your internal emotional support system. It helps you accept yourself as you are, warts and all.

When you practice self-compassion, you're setting the stage for self-forgiveness. You lower the defenses you've built to protect against the harsh critic inside your head. With self-compassion, you start seeing yourself in a new light—one that focuses on **growth** rather than punishment. This new perspective can be incredibly freeing. Imagine it like peeling layers of an onion. Each layer you let go of brings you closer to the core, to your true self.

One way to put all this into practice is through a "Self-Forgiveness Ritual." It's a simple, empowering technique. Find a quiet spot and sit down—maybe with a pen and paper. Jot down the things that are bugging you; those nagging thoughts you can't shake. Write them out. Sometimes seeing them in black and white makes them less scary.

Next, read them aloud to yourself. Acknowledge each item on your list. Now, say out loud, "I forgive myself for..." and fill in the blank with each thing you wrote down. It might feel weird at first, but stick with it—it can be really powerful. As you do this, imagine each thing blowing away like leaves in the wind.

Another step is to mentally revisit the scene of the mistake. Picture it with yourself in a more compassionate light. Replace the harsh judgment with understanding. Realize that you did what you did based on what you knew then. And that person who made the mistake? They've grown since then. They're not you anymore.

You can also close this ritual with a symbolic gesture. Maybe burn the piece of paper you wrote on. Or, if fire isn't safe or practical, tear it up and throw it away. The act of letting it go physically can help you do so emotionally.

Practicing self-forgiveness isn't a one-and-done deal. It's a continuous **process**. Just like you wouldn't do one workout and claim to be fit forever. Every time self-blame sneaks back in, remind yourself of this ritual—it's your personal self-forgiveness toolkit.

Hey, we've all been there. It's not easy, but oh—is it worth it. Finding that inner **peace** is like finally putting down that heavy bag and taking a clear, deep breath.

Moving Forward After Forgiveness

When you're in that incredible space where you've **forgiven** someone, how do you keep it up without setting yourself up for another punch in the gut? It's tricky, but stick with me. Keeping a forgiving mindset, believe it or not, doesn't mean you're a doormat. It means you've learned to let go of the past without letting people walk all over you. Here's the trick: forgiveness is for you, not for them. Always think of it that way.

Think about it like this. If someone hurt you once, you don't have to keep walking into their fists. Forgiving them clears away the emotional junk, but it doesn't mean inviting more chaos into your life. You can keep your **heart** open without leaving yourself exposed. It's like the difference between having an open window to let in fresh air and leaving your front door wide open for strangers to waltz in anytime they want.

Setting **boundaries** after you've forgiven someone is key. They're your go-to tool for making sure you don't end up back in the same mess. It's like putting up a fence around your garden; you're not stopping the rain and sun from reaching your plants, just keeping out the weeds and pests. When you set boundaries, you're saying, "Hey, I'm cool with forgiving you, but I'm not okay with you hurting me again."

Boundaries aren't as scary as they sound. Maybe it's telling a friend who once spread rumors about you how you prefer to share things in confidence. Or maybe it's deciding that time alone is sacred because you need space to heal. Whatever it is, boundaries are a way of teaching people how to treat you. And they help you stay mentally **healthy** without closing off completely. You're sort of saying, "I forgive you, but here's what's changed."

Now, let's chat about the "Lessons Learned" method. This one is perfect for finding **growth** opportunities from past hurts without dwelling on them. Think of it like mining for gold in a cave—sure, it's dark and maybe even a little damp, but there's treasure to be found that makes it worth the effort.

Start with this: What did the experience teach you about yourself? Did you find out you're stronger than you thought? Or perhaps you learned something about the kind of people you should avoid. You're like a detective, but instead of looking for clues outside, you're looking inward. Every hurt, every bump in the road has a nugget of **wisdom** hidden in it.

The best part? These lessons aren't just valuable for avoiding future pain; they're like textbooks for personal growth. For example, if you learned that you're bad at saying no, that's a huge takeaway. You can work on being more **assertive**, and guess what? You might find you get more respect from folks around you. Life's a bit like a video game—you level up with each lesson learned.

In wrapping up, moving forward after forgiveness isn't as mystical as it sounds. It's nothing more than learning to stand up for yourself while keeping your heart open. With forgiveness, boundaries, and a bit of introspection, you'll find you're not just surviving but honestly **thriving**.

Practical Exercise: Forgiveness Letter

Let's talk about writing a **forgiveness** letter. It might sound a bit heavy, but it's all about your peace of mind. Here's how you can break it down into manageable chunks.

First, pick someone or a situation you want to forgive. Think of a person who's hurt you or a situation that still **haunts** you. It could be a friend who betrayed you, a boss who dismissed you unfairly, or even yourself for past mistakes. Choose something that still stings a bit.

Next, write a letter sharing your **feelings** about the hurt or wrong. Don't sweat it; no one's grading you. Pour it all out like you're having a heart-to-heart with a friend. Let the words flow, and be honest about how this thing or person made you feel. Use everyday language, nothing fancy. "When you did X, I felt Y" is enough. Just get it all out there.

Now, recognize how this experience has **affected** your life. Sure, it can be tough, but this is important. Write down the ripple effects. Has it made you less trusting? Did it mess with your confidence or happiness? Pinpoint the exact ways it has lingered in your **emotional** life.

Say that you've decided to forgive, without expecting anything in return. State it directly in your letter. "I forgive you" or "I forgive myself" are powerful words. This is you taking back your power. Forget waiting for an apology that may never come. This is your call.

Think about any lessons or personal **growth** that came from this experience. Did it make you stronger, wiser, or more aware of red flags? Write those down, too. Yeah, it sounds a bit cliché, but there's usually some silver lining in our struggles, some quiet lessons.

After that, it's all about letting go. Wrap up the letter with a statement of releasing any anger or resentment. You could say, "I let go of the resentment I've held onto," or something that feels right to you. Visualize the hurt floating away, like you're setting a balloon free.

Finally, choose whether to send the letter or do a personal act of letting go, like burning it. If it's appropriate and safe, you might want to send the letter. Sometimes sharing it brings **closure**. But if that's not possible, burning it, burying it, or shredding it can be incredibly therapeutic. Think of this as the last step in cutting ties with that old hurt.

This exercise might seem odd at first, but sticking through it can release those **emotional** weights you're carrying around. So, grab a pen, find some quiet, and give yourself the gift of forgiveness.

In Conclusion

Forgiveness can be a tricky business, but it's incredibly important for your inner peace and happiness. This chapter helps you understand why forgiveness matters and gives you steps to begin the process. It's like **cleaning** out a mental space so you can feel lighter and freer.

In this chapter, you've learned about the true **meaning** of forgiveness and how it's different from just saying someone didn't do something wrong. You've discovered how forgiving helps you more than it helps the person you're forgiving, making your heart and mind healthier.

You've been introduced to the "Four Ds" (**Decide**, Deepen, Do, Deepen Again) that guide you on how to forgive effectively. You've also learned the difference between forgiving yourself and just excusing your bad behaviors.

The chapter has provided you with practical **steps**, like writing a "Forgiveness Letter," to help you start forgiving. It's all about taking what you've learned and applying it to your daily life. **Forgiveness** may not be easy, but with patience and practice, you can reclaim your peace and **happiness**.

Remember, it's not about letting someone off the hook; it's about freeing yourself from the burden of holding onto grudges. As you close this chapter, think about how you can take small **steps** to let go of bitterness. By doing so, you'll open your heart to more joy and love.

So, why not give it a shot? Start small, be patient with yourself, and watch how forgiveness can **transform** your life. It's time to lighten your load and embrace a more peaceful you.

Chapter 13: Perspective-Taking for Emotional Freedom

Ever **wondered** why some folks can keep cool in heated moments and sort out issues with ease? Well, I did too, until I stumbled upon something that totally changed the game—**perspective-taking**. You know those times when **emotions** run hot, and arguments feel like battles? By shifting how you see things, you're not just avoiding fights, you're actually defusing them—and coming out stronger on the other side.

Think about the last time you got into a quarrel. You probably wanted the other person to see things your way, right? In this chapter, we're diving into how flipping **viewpoints** can ease tension. By doing this, you'll start noticing that instead of getting mad, you'll start feeling more at peace. It's like having a secret **superpower** to zap out resentment.

But it doesn't stop there. Perspective-taking does wonders for your **emotional** smarts. Imagine understanding where folks are coming from without turning into a mess yourself. Practicing this **skill** bit by bit can really up your empathy game—nifty, huh? Plus, there's a neat practical **exercise** thrown in at the end, giving you a hands-on way to start this magical transformation today. Keep reading, and let's see where this goes.

Developing Empathy and Understanding

Ever wonder why some people seem to **understand** others effortlessly? It's empathy. But there's more to it. It's like empathy has two sides – thinking empathy and feeling empathy.

Thinking empathy is when you can grasp someone's situation with your head. You get the logic and facts of what's happening to them. You sort of "grok" their struggles but don't really feel them. You know how when you're listening to someone talk about their problems and you're nodding along, getting the gist? That's thinking empathy at work.

But feeling empathy goes way deeper. It's when you actually **feel** in your gut what the other person is going through. Your emotions sync with theirs. Ever watch a sad movie and cried even though you knew it's just a story? That's feeling empathy. You're connecting to someone's emotions, not just their situation.

Now, let's talk about why it matters. Feeling empathy can be a game-changer for your **stress** levels. Seriously. When you really get someone's emotions and walk a mile in their shoes, you start to see why they might be acting a certain way. This understanding makes things less personal and stressful. You realize it's not all about you. Liberating in a sense. It's almost like a weight lifted off your shoulders because you're seeing through someone else's lens for a while.

And the long-term impact on **relationships**? Huge. When you connect with others on a feeling level, it's like magic for building trust and closeness. People are drawn to those who truly "get" them. They open up more, making connections stronger and more real. You can't underestimate the energy in relationships when there's an empathy boost.

149

So, how do you get better at feeling empathy? Start with **listening**. Really listening. Not just hearing someone and waiting for your turn to talk. It's harder than it sounds in our fast-paced chatterbox world. But slowing down and giving someone your full attention can be a radical act.

Think about a time when someone really listened to you. They probably did a few key things: maintained eye contact, nodded along, and threw in a few "I see" or "I understand" to keep you talking. They didn't interrupt or steer the conversation back to themselves. Instead, they stayed present with you, making you feel heard. It felt good, right? That's what you aim for when practicing feeling empathy.

Sometimes, you can show you're engaged by repeating back what the person said in your own words. Not in a robotic way but enough to let them know you took in what they said. Something like, "So, sounds like you're saying that work's been a real grind lately…" can go a long way. It's **validating** for the person speaking and gives you a chance to really internalize their experience.

Learning to pick up on non-verbal cues also helps. People's facial expressions, body language, tones of voice – they're all pieces of the puzzle of how they feel. When you see someone with their arms crossed and a scowl, it's clear they might be upset or defensive. Let those signs fill in the gaps their words might leave out.

Small everyday **practice** makes perfect. Put away your phone when someone's talking to you. Nod along and make eye contact. Reflect back bits of what you heard to make sure you got it. Soon enough, feeling empathy will become second nature, lowering your stress and deepening all those **connections** in your life. Go on and give it a try.

Shifting Viewpoints in Conflicts

Conflicts can feel like they trap you in a corner, right? But what if I told you that shifting how you view the argument could free you? Here's where cognitive reappraisal steps in. Fancy name for a pretty simple idea. It means you take a step back and **rethink** how you see the situation, changing your initial emotional response to something more useful.

Imagine you're having a heated **argument** with your friend over a missed event. Instead of sticking to the same point and getting angrier, you try to see things differently. Maybe your friend had something unexpected come up, or perhaps they truly forgot. When you shift your viewpoint, it stops being just about your hurt feelings and opens the door to understanding. You start to see **solutions** rather than walls.

Viewing things from different angles isn't just about cooling tempers, though. It can get your creative juices flowing when finding ways out of a dispute. Have you ever noticed that some of the best ideas come when you're not stuck on one track? For instance, you and a colleague might argue about how to approach a shared project. By viewing the situation from their **perspective**, you might realize there's a hybrid solution that combines both your thoughts in a way that works even better. This kind of thinking breaks the gridlock and helps you arrive at something neither of you could have come up with alone.

So, how do you get into the practice of looking at things from these different angles? That's where the "Perspective Rotation" technique comes into play. It's a systematic way to explore various viewpoints in a **conflict**. Think of it as turning a Rubik's cube—each twist and turn you make lets you see a different color, a new angle. Here's how it works:

• **Pause** and Reflect: When a conflict arises, hit the mental pause button. Take a few deep breaths and calm down. Seriously, raging emotions won't help anyone.

• Identify Viewpoints: Break down the situation into the different viewpoints involved. Yours, theirs, and maybe even a third-party perspective if it fits.

• Step Into Their Shoes: Try to see the situation from the other party's point of view. Not easy, but incredibly worth it. Ask yourself why they might be feeling or acting the way they are.

• Compare Notes: Think about the differences in these perspectives. What's the overlap? What's totally opposite? This comparison can reveal surprising insights.

• Find Common Ground: Use these insights to identify a middle ground. Solutions that make everyone happy start to emerge here. It's all about balancing the needs and preferences discovered in each viewpoint.

You're conditioned to think your version of reality is the 'right' one. It takes practice to keep turning that Rubik's cube, especially when you're emotionally charged. But with time, this technique becomes a reliable way to clear the fog and see the real issues — and the paths out.

Staying stuck in one view is like wearing blinders. You miss out on possibilities and **solutions**. But shift your perspective, and suddenly, new doors open up. You're not just talking back and forth at each other, you're working together towards understanding and, ultimately, **resolution**. There's emotional freedom in that, a kind of lightness that comes from not being bogged down.

So, think of "Perspective Rotation" as your handy toolkit for the next conflict. Give it a whirl—twist and turn until you find those aligning colors and create the full picture.

Reducing Resentment Through Perspective

You've probably had moments where **resentment** stuck to you like gum on a shoe. Broadening your viewpoint can really help lessen that bad feeling. When you're wrapped up in resentment, it's tough to see things clearly. A broader **perspective** helps you step back and maybe even realize things aren't as bad as they seemed.

Let's talk about how to do this. Imagine looking at a situation from different angles, almost like turning a kaleidoscope. You get so many new patterns, right? Maybe that person who annoyed you had no idea they did something hurtful. Or perhaps they were dealing with their own pile of stress, making them act out without meaning to. By widening your perspective, you're more likely to spot these nuances and understand the whole picture better.

Next up is something called "fundamental attribution error." It's a psychological trick our minds play on us that keeps resentment going. This idea means that we tend to blame other people's actions on their character flaws. If someone's late, you might instantly think they're lazy. However, if you're late, you blame traffic or a late start at home. Funny how that works, huh? This habit of misjudging can really power **resentment**. You're quick to think the worst of others while cutting yourself plenty of slack.

By catching yourself in this mental trap, you can start to see things more honestly. Are you mad because someone messed up, or are you just caught in this attribution error? Being aware of this tendency gives you the chance to ask better questions and find better answers. Instead of assuming someone's rude, think they might just be having a rough time. This can make it easier to let go of resentment.

Here's a little **exercise** to try: Charitable Interpretation. This exercise is like mental yoga for assuming good intentions. Say someone cut you off in traffic—annoying, right? Instead of boiling over in anger, try thinking about non-bad reasons they might've done that. Maybe they didn't see you, or they're rushing to the hospital. Giving them the benefit of the doubt takes the sting out.

If you want to practice this in another setting, take a situation where you felt wronged and try putting yourself in the other person's shoes. What might they have been thinking? What pressures could they have been under? It's not about making excuses; it's about choosing a less bad viewpoint that allows you to move on without holding onto that heavy bag of resentment.

Practicing charitable interpretations can also improve your **relationships**. Once others sense you're willing to give them a break, they're often more understanding with you. Everybody wins a bit here. You get to drop the anger, and your interactions become smoother.

So, stretch your perspective. Catch yourself when you're falling into the fundamental attribution error. Practice charitable interpretations. By using these **tactics**, you'll find that resentment won't stand a chance!

Now that wasn't so heavy, was it? These little shifts can make a world of difference. You might feel the release of that emotional weight. A lighter heart, clearer **mind**, and hey – fewer grudges. Life's tough enough without dragging old resentments around. Give these approaches a shot, and watch how they change not just your inner world but how you **connect** with everyone around you.

Enhancing Emotional Intelligence

It's crucial to **see** things from another person's perspective. This can really help you understand and handle **emotions** better. For instance, when you're in a heated argument with someone, pausing to consider why they're upset can make it easier to calm down and deal with the situation. Imagine trying to address an angry customer. If you understand they've probably had a bad day or a frustrating experience, their anger starts making more sense. Recognizing their emotional state helps you respond in a supportive way. It's all about walking a mile in their shoes, and it's incredibly handy in all kinds of relationships.

Thinking about social thinking is key too. It's about figuring out what's going on in other people's heads and why they **act** the way they do. Have you ever noticed how some folks seem to just know what to say or do in tricky social situations? They're like mind readers. That's social thinking at work. They pick up on little hints, like tone of voice or body language, and make a guess about what someone else is feeling or thinking. It's not always spot-on, but just the effort to understand can make a huge difference. It makes social stuff less awkward, and you don't feel so out of place at a gathering or meeting.

Speaking of which, how do you get better at spotting these clues? Here's where the "Emotion Mapping" trick comes into play. It's a simple **exercise** that helps you notice what others are feeling and guess why. Start by watching people's faces when they talk. Notice the way their eyes move, how they smile, or if they frown. Combine this with what they're saying and how they're saying it. Jot down your thoughts later if it helps. Say your buddy seems distant; connect that by thinking, "Hey, maybe they had a tough day at work." Over time, you'll get more accurate at judging these emotions, almost like your own emotional radar.

For a fun practice, think back to a recent **conversation**. Make a list in your mind or on paper: what words did they use, what were their facial expressions, and what could those mean about their feelings? The key here is practice and patience.

Learning these tricks is like unlocking another level in a game. Each time you get a bit better, everything gets just a bit easier. Whether it's small talk at a party, understanding your boss's critique, or helping a friend through a rough patch, you'll find the pieces start to click into place. They suddenly make more sense. It helps you see another side of the story and makes your responses more caring and less reactive. Less chance they say "You're not listening," and more real **connection**.

Emotional **intelligence** isn't just about knowing emotions. It's about seeing them, in yourself and others, and figuring out the best way to handle them. Master this and you're playing life on hard mode with cheat codes. **Communication** becomes clearer, **relationships** stronger and, let's face it, life gets a bit smoother and a lot more satisfying. Stick with it; it's rewarding beyond belief.

Practical Exercise: Perspective-Shifting

You're dealing with some sort of **conflict** or misunderstanding, right? Uh-oh. Just pick one that's been hanging around in your mind lately. Might be with a friend, coworker, family member—it doesn't really matter. The point is, it's bugging you. Got it? Good.

Next up, grab a piece of paper or open your notes app. Jot down how you see the situation. Doesn't have to be fancy—just your feelings and assumptions. Why do you think things got messed up? What's been said or done that ticks you off? Be honest with yourself here. Lay it all out there because this is your truth according to you. Keep it casual, like you're telling a friend.

Now, picture yourself as the other person in this situation. Flip the script. Try to really get into their shoes, like you're an actor in a movie. What might they be feeling? What **assumptions** might they be making about you? Write this down too, pretending you are them. Channel your inner method actor, if you catch my drift. This perspective-shifting thing can be quite the eye-opener.

Here comes the tricky part, but stick with me. Think like a fly on the wall—a neutral third party. Someone who doesn't have a dog in this fight. Describe what's going on, but do it objectively. No emotions, no bias. Just the facts, ma'am. What happened from a purely neutral stance? Pretend you're writing a news article—keep it straightforward and factual. This will feel weird after writing all the emotional stuff, but it's kinda crucial.

Now it's time for **reflection**. Look over what you've written from each of these perspectives. Chew on it for a bit. What's new here? Did you learn something surprising about yourself or the other person? Sometimes just seeing it all laid out can shift your mindset in ways you didn't expect.

With these variances of insight, start looking at **solutions**. Yeah, fixing stuff comes after understanding it from all angles. Think of potential ways to resolve the issue that considers everyone's worries and needs. Write out a few ideas, no matter how simple or complex. Practical works. No need for some grand peace treaty—just stuff you might actually do.

And finally, roll out your **action** plan. Look at your possible solutions and pick one or two that seem feasible. Flesh out a simple plan on how to approach the person and work on patching things up. Timing matters, so think about the right setting, the right words, the right time. It's about putting yourself in their shoes and figuring out how you'd wanna be addressed if the tables were turned.

Perspective-Shifting isn't a magic wand, but it's close. It teaches you to look at the bigger **picture**. Next time you're stuck in your head, guiding yourself through these steps can unlock the combo to healthier **interactions**—you might just solve some of those nagging **conflicts** hanging over your best moments.

In Conclusion

In this chapter, you've discovered the **importance** of perspective-taking for achieving emotional freedom. By looking at situations from different viewpoints, you can better **understand** yourself and others, leading to more harmonious relationships and personal growth. Here's a quick rundown:

You've learned about the difference between cognitive and emotional empathy and how they help in understanding others' feelings. You've seen how developing empathy can reduce your own stress and make friendships stronger. You've also explored practicing active listening as a core skill to become more empathetic.

You've delved into using cognitive reappraisal in conflicts to keep your cool and solve problems more creatively. Plus, you've learned about the "Perspective Rotation" technique to **resolve** conflicts effectively by exploring different viewpoints.

Applying these **insights** can make you emotionally aware and capable of handling challenging situations with ease. Start practicing perspective-taking every day, and you'll notice a positive **change** in how you connect with others and manage your emotions.

Keep these concepts in mind and try to apply them to your daily **experiences**. You have the power to improve your relationships and bring more peace into your life through empathy and perspective-taking. Keep at it, and you'll see the **difference**!

Remember, it's all about putting yourself in someone else's shoes. The more you **practice**, the better you'll get at navigating tricky social situations and keeping your cool when things get heated. So go ahead, give it a shot, and watch how it transforms your interactions and your overall outlook on life!

To Conclude

The **essence** of this book lies in its title: offering you practical techniques to stop **ruminating** on the past, heal emotionally, and enjoy the freedom that's rightfully yours. It's about shifting from a state of overthinking and emotional entanglement to one of **peace** and proactive living. You've been on a transformative journey, learning how to let go and fully **engage** with the present.

Here's a quick recap. We dove into the psychological aspects of letting go, understanding how emotions play a crucial role and that recognizing overthinking patterns is the first step to breaking free. You learned about emotional **intelligence** and self-awareness, realizing that unresolved experiences impact your overall well-being. Building resilience through self-compassion and understanding the mind-body connection were other key points.

We talked about the dichotomy of control. By learning to distinguish between controllable and uncontrollable factors, you can focus your **energy** on actionable areas and accept what can't be changed. Mastering nonjudgmental awareness helps you reduce stress and enhance emotional regulation by observing thoughts without attachment.

The techniques we covered enabled you to create psychological space from your emotions for better perspective and reduced emotional intensity. We addressed breaking the chains of negativity, revealing how overcoming self-defeating behaviors can foster a positive mindset. Adopting a growth mindset helps you see challenges as opportunities and develop **resilience** and adaptability.

We focused on silencing the inner critic by identifying and challenging negative self-talk patterns, ultimately leading to stronger self-compassion. You learned about the pitfalls of perfectionism and how adopting a more growth-oriented mindset supports setting realistic and healthy standards without self-judgment.

We then moved onto the practice of nonattachment, describing how letting go of outcomes and expectations develops emotional flexibility. Techniques for rewriting negative self-scripts reinforce the constructive narratives you tell yourself. We also spoke about the importance of **forgiveness**, for both others and yourself, as a pathway to inner peace. Perspective-taking for emotional freedom was emphasized, encouraging empathy and shifting viewpoints to reduce resentment.

So, what's next? Imagine a life where you've mastered these techniques—letting go of past hurts effortlessly, approaching life's challenges with a proactive mindset, and experiencing true emotional freedom. The principles in this book aren't just tips; they're life-altering practices that can redefine how you experience your world.

Take these insights to heart and apply them diligently. The road ahead may have its bumps, but equipped with these tools, you're ready to face them with resilience and grace.

Visit this link to find out more:

https://pxl.to/LoganMind

Other Books

When it comes to **personal growth** and true emotional well-being, expanding your knowledge beyond one topic is essential. This book has provided you valuable techniques for letting go, but complementing it with related subjects will deepen your understanding and effectiveness. I have authored a series of books—either available now or about to be released—that delve into themes crucial to emotional health and resilience.

Next up is **Emotional Agility**, where you'll learn how to adapt and respond more effectively to life's changes. It teaches you mental flexibility and how to handle stress and uncertainty, something you'll grapple with at various stages. Imagine coupling the power of letting go with a newfound ability to pivot gracefully in any scenario.

My subsequent book, **Emotional Burnout**, targets the inevitable wear and tear your mind experiences. Many focus only on the symptoms, but I get into the root causes and how to rejuvenate your emotional fuel before it runs out. Think of the power in combining the art of letting go with strategies to prevent and heal inner exhaustion.

Lastly, **Emotional Stability** presents foundational pillars to achieve lasting balance in your emotional life. While learning to let go is transformative, maintaining equilibrium ensures this newfound peace remains. This resource is invaluable if you're looking to sustain long-term emotional health.

To dig deeper and expand on what you've learned, here's what you can do:

• Check out the link below

• Click on "All My Books"

• Grab the ones that catch your eye

• If you want to get in touch with me, you'll find all the contact info at the end of the link

Check out all my books and contacts here:

https://pxl.to/LoganMind

Help Me!

When you support an independent author, you're supporting a dream.

If you're **satisfied** with my work, why not leave an **honest** review by clicking the link below? Your opinion is **gold**, and it can shape not just my future books but other readers' experiences too.

Got some ideas for **improvements**? Shoot me an email using the contact info at the link below. Your constructive criticism is like fuel for my growth as a writer.

Or if you're feeling techy, you can **scan** the QR code and find the link after picking your book.

It'll only take a few seconds, but your **voice** packs a huge punch.

Your feedback is a real **treasure** that can light a fire under my writing journey. Together, we can keep churning out **amazing** stories and experiences.

Check out this link to leave your thoughts:

https://pxl.to/7-tpolg-lm-review

Join my Review Team!

Thank you so much for reading my book. Your **support** means the world to me, and I'd love to invite you to be part of my **Review** team. If you're an avid **reader**, you can receive a free copy of my book in exchange for an honest **review**. Your **feedback** is invaluable and helps me improve with each new release.

Here's how you can join the ARC team:

• Click on the link or scan the QR code.

• Click on the book cover on the page that opens up.

• Click on "Join Review Team."

• Sign up to BookSprout.

• Get notified every time I release a new **book**.

Your **involvement** in this process is super easy and straightforward. By joining, you'll not only get your hands on free books but also play a crucial role in shaping future **releases**. It's a win-win situation where you get to indulge in your passion for reading while helping an author grow.

Check out the team here:

https://pxl.to/loganmindteam

Don't miss this chance to become part of an exciting literary journey!